20 YEARS YOUNGER

ALSO BY BOB GREENE

The Life You Want: Get Motivated, Lose Weight, and Be Happy

The Best Life Diet

Bob Greene's Total Body Makeover

Get With the Program!

Make the Connection: Ten Steps to a Better Body — and a Better Life

Keep the Connection: Choices for a Better Body and a Better Life

20 YEARS YOUNGER

Look Younger, Feel Younger, Be Younger!

BOB GREENE

with Harold A. Lancer, MD, Ronald L. Kotler, MD, and Diane L. McKay, PhD

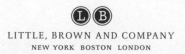

LITTLE, BROWN AND COMPANY
NEW YORK BOSTON LONDON

Little, Brown and Company
Hachette Book Group
237 Park Avenue, New York, NY 10017
www.hachettebookgroup.com

First Edition: April 2011

Little, Brown and Company is a division of Hachette Book Group, Inc. The Little, Brown name and logo are trademarks of Hachette Book Group, Inc.

This book is intended to supplement, not replace, the advice of a trained health professional. Before starting a diet plan, or beginning or modifying an exercise program, check with your physician to make sure that the changes are appropriate for you. If you know or suspect that you have a health problem, you should consult a health professional. The author and publisher specifically disclaim any liability, loss, or risk, personal or otherwise, which is incurred as a consequence, directly or indirectly, of the use and application of any of the contents of this book.

The publisher is not responsible for websites (or their content) that are not owned by the publisher.

Illustrations by Molly Borman-Pullen

Library of Congress Cataloging-in-Publication Data
Greene, Bob.
    20 years younger : look younger, feel younger, be younger! / Bob Greene ; with Harold Lancer, Ronald L. Kotler, and Diane L. McKay.
        p. cm.
    ISBN 978-0-316-13378-4 (hc) / 978-0-316-17796-2 (large print)
    1. Longevity.   I. Lancer, Harold.   II. Kotler, Ronald L.   III. McKay, Diane L.
IV. Title.
    RA776.75.G74 2011
    613.2 — dc22   2010048827

10 9 8 7 6 5 4 3 2 1

RRD-C

Printed in the United States of America

Contents

20 YEARS YOUNGER

Introduction

SEVERAL YEARS AGO, I spent part of the spring cycling my way across the country, riding from Long Beach, California, to New York City. It was something I had always wanted to do, and the opportunity presented itself when I was booked on a multicity tour to promote a book I'd written. I knew that the 3,600-mile trip would be grueling, but I thought it would actually be less stressful than racing from one airport to another, which is how a typical book tour unfolds. To prepare, I trained hard so that I'd be able to hit my target of riding about one hundred miles a day. I planned to sleep in a different town every night and visit bookstores, malls, and fitness centers in more than thirty cities along the way.

I wasn't far into the trip when I began to feel dramatic changes taking place. By the time I hit Arizona, I had a mental and emotional clarity that I'd never before experienced. At times, I'd be riding for eight hours or more with nothing but the sound of my own breathing and the beat of my heart in my ears. As I looked around me, colors seemed brighter, the world smelled fresher, sounds seemed sharper, the things I touched seemed more textured. All my senses were amplified. And nothing rattled me — not a dog giving chase, rain on my back, a treacherous ascent. As my legs cycled rhythmically, the pedestrian concerns of the everyday slipped away and I'd find my thinking stripped down to the essentials. I contemplated the scenery and I contemplated my life. What was important to me? What did I want out of life? While I was on that trip it all became so much clearer.

As I edged toward Chicago I became aware that I was also going through extraordinary physical changes. I'd been hailed on at the Grand Canyon and twice climbed more than 11,000 feet in the still snowy Rockies, and I felt invincible, virtually bulletproof. Every night I slept like a rock. In my early forties at the time, I thought I was pretty fit going into the ride, but that extreme physical challenge left me much stronger than I'd ever been in my life, even in my twenties.

While I knew riding cross-country would be a challenge and that I'd come off the bike fitter than when I started, I hadn't realized how much the trip would transform me both physically and emotionally. I was particularly amazed at how clearheaded I felt. I was able to look at my life and see exactly where I wanted to go. By the time I reached the East Coast, I was operating on all cylinders and had regained (and even significantly surpassed) the strength, power, energy, lucidity, and drive of my earlier years.

Graduate students in exercise physiology learn about the anti-aging benefits of physical activity, and I was no exception. In fact, I'd had a longtime interest in the science of aging and the prevention of age-related decline. But once my cross-country trip allowed me to see the possibilities for myself, I became passionate about the subject. It wasn't long after I completed that cross-country tour that I started exploring ideas for this book.

It's not practical for most people to get on a bike and ride for a month (it's not something I could easily fit into my life anymore either), but I wondered if there were adjustments you could make to your everyday life that would have a similar de-aging, life-enhancing effect. I knew that a good fitness plan could go a long way toward turning back the clock, but what else was possible? To find out, I spent the next few years talking to experts in other fields, learning about the latest advances in anti-aging science and determining what aspects of that research could be translated into a workable plan for daily life.

After a time, it became evident that there are four main fronts on which you can vigorously fight back against the effects of aging: exercise, nutrition, skin care, and restorative sleep. Addressing any one of these areas with an eye toward shaving off the years can have a tremendous payoff, but it pales in comparison to the combined impact of all four—especially when you also control the stress in your life and practice positive thinking, two other aspects that can significantly slow the aging process. A well-rounded comprehensive approach can not only help you look and feel younger, but can actually make your body reverse course, even at the cellular level. At this point there's little doubt: Good anti-aging strategies can both extend your life *and* substantially raise the quality of it.

By calling this book *20 Years Younger* I'm making what some might think is an exaggerated claim. But most people these days are living lives that predispose them to early aging. If you grab ahold of your health and actively pursue greater well-being, I don't think it's extravagant to say that you can dramatically turn things around. It's commonly accepted that the body undergoes certain changes with age, and to some extent those changes are inevitable. Even works of art maintained under pristine light and temperature conditions eventually begin to wither. What is less known, though, is that the life you lead and the decisions you make every day are largely responsible for how quickly, profoundly, and noticeably you age. In fact, much of what we think of as aging—wrinkles, weight gain, memory loss, lack of energy, certain types of illnesses—is not primarily attributable to the passage of time. Rather, it's a direct result of sedentary living, poor diet, lack of sleep, insufficient (or nonexistent) skin care, too much stress, and even a defeatist attitude. It stands to reason, then, that if you reverse those habits— if you get moving, eat longevity-promoting foods, sleep soundly and adequately, protect and nourish your skin, and improve your outlook on the world—the signs of aging will reverse themselves, too.

Some people *have* gotten the message that the life you lead can indeed turn back the clock. But I feel others have misinterpreted the message to mean that they should zealously pursue any program that promises everlasting youth. Extreme exercise regimens, severely restrictive diets, unproven hormonal therapies, cosmetic surgery makeovers—they may all seem like quick and effective ways to return the body to its youthful self, but more often than not they're counterproductive. What we're offering you in this book instead are natural, research-based strategies for getting your body (and mind) in top form and even lowering your physiological age. The goal isn't to help you turn yourself back into a teenager but rather to help you lead your longest, fullest, and healthiest life. Stay strong, energetic, mentally sharp, and confident, and your age will not define—or debilitate—you. Instead it will be incidental; something noted on your driver's license but not indicative of your health or capabilities.

I'm in my fifties now and I've always prided myself in trying to live a healthy life. Some of those habits, as it turns out, have helped me when it comes to aging. I've been extremely conscientious about exercise, of course, and I'd give myself a pretty good grade in healthy eating, getting enough sleep, and controlling stress, too. The one area where I wish I'd been more diligent is in caring for my skin. It's long been my Achilles' heel.

Like so many people, I grew up before the widespread use of sunscreen. Nobody had heard of SPF back then, and while we knew that getting sunburn hurt, we hadn't been clued in to the dangers of sun exposure. I've always had rather fair skin, and when a friend of mine in my elementary school suggested I get a tan, I began to feel self-conscious about how pale I was—an insecurity that lingered well into early adulthood. I never was that successful at getting a tan (I always burned instead), but that doesn't mean I didn't try.

A number of years ago Oprah and I were training for a race when, probably annoyed at me for urging her to "push harder," she turned to me and said, "I've never met anyone so together. Is there anything you struggle with?" "Well, I don't tan very well," I replied, giving an honest answer. Oprah burst out laughing. I know she thought I was kidding, but I was genuinely insecure about my fair skin!

As I gathered information for this book and went looking for an expert to contribute a chapter on skin care, I thought I might be able to use myself as a guinea pig. By now I was regretting every unprotected minute I'd spent in the sun, and I needed some help in rejuvenating my skin. My plan was to interview several top-echelon dermatologists, try their products and advice, and see how well they — and I — fared.

By the time I met Harold A. Lancer, MD, I'd already talked to a few different doctors and tried their plans, but with less than stellar results. When I went in to see Dr. Lancer, both his knowledge and his demeanor immediately impressed me. During my appointment, he had me take off my shirt so he could assess the skin below my chin, and then he proceeded to call in his staff of assistants and nurses. There I was, with a group of women looking at me as if I were in a petri dish, when Dr. Lancer said, "Look at him. He has the body of someone decades younger." Just when I was starting to feel a little puffed up, he added, "His skin, though — that's just about right for his age." He started to point out all my sun damage and age spots. I was hoping for a better report, but given that I have the kind of skin that wrinkles if you look at it too long, I wasn't surprised. And Dr. Lancer, as you'll see when you read his chapter, tells it like it is.

What I like most about Dr. Lancer's approach (and I think you will, too) is that he has shown that you can get your skin to behave younger — not just look younger, but actually be younger — with three simple skin care steps. To his mind, all the popular cosmetic procedures, ranging from lasers and fillers to neurotoxins, are really beautifiers of the last resort. He sees the trend starting to go away from these more invasive interventions and toward a more cost-effective, natural, do-it-yourself approach to skin maintenance. I can say from personal experience that it really works.

Another expert whose contribution to this book offers great benefits is Ronald L. Kotler, MD. Dr. Kotler and I met when we happened to be appearing on *Good Morning America* on the same day. I watched his segment on sleep and admired his approach to getting a good night's slumber and the user-friendly way he conveyed the information. In his chapter, Dr. Kotler, who is also the coauthor, with Maryann Karinch, of *365 Ways to Get a Good Night's Sleep*, explains how sleep changes as you get older and how you can offset those changes with some simple strategies. It turns out that adequate sleep not only affects the way you look and feel but is also connected to lowering the risk of many life-shortening diseases.

I like to keep my website updated with the latest information about health, exercise, skin care, and nutrition, including vitamin, mineral, and other dietary supplements. But I'd been feeling frustrated by the quality of the supplements on the market as well as the information supporting them. They always seemed to have too much of one thing and too little of something else. I was so disappointed by what I found out there that I started thinking about developing my own line. That's when I met Diane L. McKay, PhD, to whom I turned for advice on both the efficacy and safety of supplements. Dr. McKay has done extensive research on vitamin and mineral supplementation, is up on the latest studies, and brings a bit of sanity to a topic that can be confusing and somewhat controversial. Her contributions to the book have been invaluable. In chapter 3, Dr. McKay helps separate the supplements that have true anti-aging and overall health benefits from the ones that are a waste of money, and she provides a guide to safely adding supplements to your diet.

———————————

Someone once asked Woody Allen how he felt about the aging process, and Allen answered, "Well, I'm against it." I laughed when I read that and thought to myself, *Me too!* But the truth is, I'm not really against aging. I'm simply for aging well. Accepting that you're growing older is not the same thing as accepting a life that's limited by age-related maladies or where you don't look or feel your best. Age, as they say, really *is* just a number. It's how well you're able to live your life that counts. Another showbiz guy, the comedian George Burns, once said, "You can't help getting older, but you don't have to get old." And Burns knew what he was talking about. He lived a vigorous life until the age of one hundred.

I'd like to live to one hundred, too, as long as I could still live a high-quality life at that advanced age. I'm sure most people would, but as the father of two young children, I have a particular reason for wanting to live long and have the strength and vitality to enjoy my family for many years to come. I came late to fatherhood — I was almost fifty when we had our first child — and it's given me incredible incentive to stay as energetic, healthy, and youthful as I can. If I've learned anything during the time I've spent exploring the aging process, it's that motivation is key, just as it is for achieving anything worthwhile. You can't be complacent if you want to age gracefully. It takes some discipline and hard work to slow down aging — if it were easy everyone would look and feel twenty years younger. When you commit yourself to all the elements of this plan — staying fit, eating right, caring for your skin, sticking to good sleep habits — you're distinguishing yourself from the crowd. And you'll be richly rewarded for your efforts. Examine your current lifestyle, readjust your schedule, direct your passion and drive toward adopting a new, healthier anti-aging lifestyle, and — trust me — you'll get amazing results.

PART I

THE ART AND SCIENCE OF AGING

CHAPTER 1

The Science of Aging

The longer I live, the more beautiful life becomes.
— Frank Lloyd Wright

EVERYONE HAS A NOTION of what it means to age. Whether it's a snapshot in your head of how your parents have slowed down or lines you see on your own face, for many people it has something to do with decline. Things not being the way they used to be. Everything less than before.

A lot of people feel that aging is about loss. And in some ways it is. "Aging is a wide range of physiological changes that make us more susceptible to death, limit our normal functions, and render us more susceptible to disease," says João Pedro de Magalhães, PhD, a researcher on the biology and genetics of aging and a lecturer at the University of Liverpool in England. I would add that the physiological changes that take place as we age can also render us more susceptible to psychological downturns. It's not uncommon for people to lose enthusiasm as they get older, disheartened by their physical deterioration and inability to live the way they used to.

Do we have to age? It's the $6 million—or maybe I should say $6 billion—question and it's one that researchers the world over are donating a lot of time and money to answering. Some scientists are even hoping to answer the inevitable next question: Do we have to die? I don't think we're all that much closer to immortality than Ponce de León was when he went searching for the fountain of youth in 1513. However, we do have a much greater understanding of the aging process. And we are living longer: Over the last one hundred and fifty years, the average life span has climbed from about age forty-five to closer to age eighty.

Living longer is important, but the ultimate goal is to live longer *and* live well into your later years. And through the science of aging we now know that it's very possible. In fact, it's become clearer that not all the effects of aging we've come to expect are inevitable, and that by making certain lifestyle choices you can dramatically slow those effects down—and maybe, in some cases, even eradicate them. We all age—that is undeniable—but your likelihood of aging poorly increases if you decide to sit back and leave well enough alone. To the contrary, take action and you'll retain your vitality, age gracefully, and, yes, have a longer, better life.

Each of the subsequent chapters in this book asks you to make certain lifestyle changes toward that goal. The reasons behind those changes will be clearer if you know a little bit about the theories of why we age and the physiological consequences of growing older.

THEORIES ON WHY WE AGE

Scientists have long debated a central question about aging: Why? Why do we age? Many of them, both past and present, fall into the evolutionary camp. In the late 1800s, a German by the name of August Weismann was one of the first to promote an evolutionary theory. He believed that we're programmed to age and die in order to make room for the younger generation, continuing the evolution and betterment of the species. You might call it planned obsolescence.

Over time, the evolutionary theory of aging has, well, evolved and other theories have risen to the fore. One, called the mutation accumulation theory, is based on the idea that undesirable genes that cause the death of children get weeded out; they're not passed on to the next generation. But undesirable genes that don't cause death until late in life get passed on from generation to generation because the people who have those genes have children before their death. Over successive generations, those genes have accumulated, predisposing people to contract diseases as they grow old, then die.

Another well-known evolutionary theory is called the antagonistic pleiotropy theory. Its central idea is that some genes may be beneficial to us in our early lives but detrimental to us as we grow older. For instance, genes that increase a woman's ability to reproduce may also ultimately lead to menopause and all the health hazards (among them, bone loss and an increased risk of heart disease) that go with it. According to the antagonistic pleiotropy theory, evolution may select for genes that favor youth because the chances that humans and other organisms will survive accidents, predators, and disease to live long lives are slim (or at least were before modern medicine).

The other major theories on why we age have less to do with evolution and more to do with the cumulative effects of damage to the body. Over the years, injury from simple wear and tear, sun damage, a poor diet, smoking, pollution, even the body's own metabolic processes, add up to promote aging and eventual death. One of the most prominent of these theories focuses on oxidative stress. Oxidative stress refers to the injury done to DNA, cells, and tissues in the body by free radicals, molecules with unpaired electrons that are produced when the body metabolizes oxygen. Free radicals also become present in the body through all the injurious means I just mentioned (poor diet, etc.). In their incomplete state, free radicals become thieves, stealing electrons from other molecules and wreaking havoc along the way. The damage they leave in their wake is often compared to the rusting of metal. The body has the ability to absorb free radicals and repair the damage they do, but its defense system tends to weaken over time, leaving it vulnerable to disease.

Like all theories about the cause of aging, the oxidative stress theory is just that, theory. We don't know for sure if unbound free radicals are the main cause of aging; however, we *do* know that free radicals cause harm and that oxidative damage can certainly age your body, decrease your quality of life, and even shorten your life span. More specifically, by damaging a cell's DNA, oxidative stress can be the first step to transforming a healthy cell into a cancer cell (cancer also has other causes, such as inherited genetic mutations). Free radicals influence LDL (bad) cholesterol as well, making it even more prone to sticking to the walls of arteries and increasing the risk of heart disease, stroke, erectile dysfunction, and other conditions.

Many of the strategies you'll read about in this book are aimed at preventing and repairing free radical damage. I'll be recommending many foods that contain antioxidants such as vitamin E, vitamin C, and certain phytonutrients that disarm and disable free radicals. These dietary watchdogs also boost the body's own free radical defense system. Likewise, the exercise program will help turn up your body's own free radical–fighting capabilities. A lot of Dr. Lancer's skin care recommendations also focus on quenching free radicals that degrade collagen and elastin, the proteins that give skin its structure and bounce.

In addition to free radicals, inflammation has been implicated in aging because of the role it plays in so many age-related diseases. (They're actually related—free radicals can cause inflammation.) Short-lived inflammation is a good thing; it's the body's defense against a flu virus, bacteria, a wound, a chemical irritant, and other kinds of trauma. Inflammation occurs when, triggered by damage, immune cells rush into the injured area, releasing compounds that destroy bacteria or promote wound healing. When the condition resolves, the immune response goes away. At least, most of the time. Sometimes, for a number of reasons, inflammation persists. That's called chronic inflammation, and it's been linked to everything from cancer and heart disease to diabetes, dementia, and even wrinkles. While it's far from certain that inflammation is the major culprit in aging, anything you can do to reduce inflammation—such as exercise regularly—will reduce the cumulative effects of aging.

In the evolutionary theory of aging, genes determine aging and, ultimately, death. In the damage theory of aging, factors such as unhealthy food, stress, and even the body's own metabolic processes are the primary agents. However, many people, including me, believe that aging is a combination of both. All the recommendations in this book, in fact, are predicated on the idea that you are working both with your own genetic predispositions and with the things in life that you can control, such as what you eat and how much you exercise. Aging without question has its foundations in genetically

The Aging Brain

Using MRI and other imaging technologies, researchers have learned that your brain starts to get smaller as you get older. "The volume of the frontal cortex, which is responsible for reasoning, problem-solving, and strategic tasks, gets smaller, and white matter gets more porous; it's not as tightly woven as it was," explains Denise Park, PhD, director of the Center for Vital Longevity in Dallas. These changes may explain why most people experience subtle declines in the rate at which they process new information, the amount of information they can process at a time, and the ability to remember new information long-term.

Memory of the past can also be affected. "As you age, it gets harder to put tags on individual memories, which allows them to be distinctive and easier to retrieve later on," says Tom Hess, PhD, professor in the department of Lifespan Developmental Psychology at North Carolina State University in Raleigh. This change in memory functioning appears to be due to age-related loss of neurons in the hippocampus, the area of the brain partially responsible for establishing new specific memories.

With age, protein deposits may start to form in the brain. The brain naturally produces a type of plaque called amyloid, which normally degrades and is eliminated by the body. Researchers have noticed a buildup of this protein during autopsies on people who had Alzheimer's disease. Up until very recently, it wasn't possible to look at plaque in healthy people, but Park and her team have been able to inject a radio tracer substance into the brain, then use imaging techniques to see whether healthy volunteers have a buildup of amyloid. They've found that between 25 and 35 percent of healthy adults start to have amyloid buildup in their forties and fifties. Park notes that the plaque is associated with some cognitive decline but that it's uncertain whether it's an early sign or stage of Alzheimer's disease. "Lots of people functioning at a high level have this plaque that's associated with Alzheimer's," she says.

Growing older isn't all bad news for the brain. Every time you learn something new, new wiring gets laid down. The result: more processing power. You can also fight the aging of the brain. Read how exercise helps on page 32, and turn to page 209 for brain-boosting tips.

determined mechanisms. "But," points out João Pedro de Magalhães, "genetics can be modulated by environmental factors."

I'll give you a good example. One of the markers of aging that you'll be hearing a lot more about in this book are telomeres. Telomeres are the tail ends of chromosomes, the structures that carry genes. Every time a cell divides, the telomeres stabilize the cell's chromosomes, but in the process they become shorter. When telomeres become too short, the cell can no longer divide and it dies. This is believed to lead to various aspects of aging, including diminished muscle strength, wrinkles, and lowered immunity. How much telomere length really affects longevity—if at all—is still unknown, but many prominent researchers believe it's an important cog in the wheel of life.

In 2008, researchers at King's College in London looked at the length of the telomeres in the white blood cells of twins. Some of the participants were very active, while their twin siblings were quite a bit less active. The results of the study showed that, across the board, telomere length was related to activity: the more active the person, the longer the telomeres. When very active exercisers were compared directly to their less active twins, they had telomere lengths that looked to be about four years younger. Here was a case where genetics were the same, but the cells were influenced by differing external factors, in this instance, exercise.

MAJOR AGING ACCELERATORS

Obesity

Being overweight predisposes the body to heart disease, but that's only one way that obesity can affect longevity and accelerate aging. New research suggests that it also makes cells older on a molecular level. For instance, some of the same researchers that looked at telomere length in active and sedentary twins also looked at telomere length in obese women. What they found was that obese women had shorter telomeres than lean women. If you translated the telomere length into years, the obese women's cells were nine years older than the lean women's. Excess body fat is also thought to cause oxidative stress and is known to promote inflammation of the kind that's been linked to age-related diseases.

Inflammation caused by excessive body fat may also be related to the shrinking of the brain. Gary Wenk, PhD, a professor of psychology, neuroscience, and molecular virology, immunology, and medical genetics at the Ohio State University and Medical Center, has shown that proteins that are a by-product of inflammation can cause regions of the brain responsible for memory and learning new things to become smaller. Other studies have shown that older people who are obese have lesser cognitive and memory capabilities and are at an increased risk for Alzheimer's disease.

Another way that obesity affects aging is by contributing to insulin resistance. Insulin is the hormone charged with ushering the sugar from your blood into cells throughout your body. When you aren't producing enough insulin, or your cells become resistant to insulin's actions, blood sugar rises. People with type 1 diabetes produce no insulin. People with type 2—the kind that is often caused by too much body fat and constitutes about 90 to 95 percent of diabetes cases—are insulin resistant. That is, their bodies don't respond properly to normal amounts of insulin so that sugar doesn't get adequately transported from the blood to the cells. People with type 2 diabetes may even eventually stop producing normal amounts of insulin, which can make the situation worse.

Insulin resistance can shorten your life span and hasten aging in a number of ways: it encourages inflammation, quashes sirtuin activity (sirtuins are enzymes that delay cell death), shortens telomeres, and raises levels of compounds called AGEs—advanced glycation end products—that wreak havoc in the body (see page 117). Besides obesity (and particularly an overabundance of intra-abdominal fat—stored fat that surrounds the organs), a diet high in sweets, sodas and other sugary drinks, white bread, white rice, and other processed grains seems to promote insulin resistance. There's a hereditary factor to insulin resistance as well—your genes may make you more susceptible. But you might be able to stave it off for longer, and if you get it, regulate your blood sugar better, with the type of diet you'll find in chapter 3.

Smoking

While the link between excessive body weight and aging is disheartening given the rates of obesity in this country, it's somewhat more surprising than what has long been known as the number one cause of preventable death: smoking. Besides its deleterious effect on life span, smoking promotes aging in just about every way imaginable. It's known, for instance, that smoking creates free radicals and that it's associated with the development of many age-related diseases, including some that you might not even think would be related: osteoporosis, diabetes, and the eye disease macular degeneration. In the obesity study I mentioned earlier, they also looked at the effect of smoking on telomeres and found that it shortened telomere length by a full 18 percent.

It's been known for some time that smoking is linked to dementia, and recently researchers at Kaiser Permanente in Oakland found that it's also associated with an increased risk of Alzheimer's disease. Compared to non-smokers, people who smoked two packs a day in midlife increased their risk of Alzheimer's by 157 percent.

Dr. Lancer will talk more about the effects of smoking on the skin in chapter 4. However, suffice it to say that there's such a thing as "smoker's face," characterized by deep lines around the mouth and eyes and a grayish tint to the skin. Nicotine contracts the blood vessels, decreasing blood flow to the skin and all the other major organs in the body.

There are a few other reasons why it's to your advantage to quit smoking. One is that it makes it difficult to exercise at the pace you need to get sizable anti-aging benefits. The other is that smoking can interfere with sleep. To see just how much, researchers at the Johns Hopkins University School of Medicine hooked up forty smokers and forty nonsmokers to monitoring machines and looked at their brain waves as they slept. The smokers spent a lot less time in deep sleep, the most rejuvenating kind of slumber, and a lot more time in the lighter stages of sleep, when it's easy to be awakened—possibly in part because they were going through nicotine withdrawal while they slept. The smokers also reported feeling less refreshed in the morning. (You'll learn more about the importance of a good night's sleep in chapter 5.) Smoking is probably the single worst thing you can do to yourself—it's like lying on a train track when you know that the train is coming. Quitting, on the other hand, is perhaps the single *best* thing you can do for yourself.

Stress

Work, finances, kids' schedules, relationship problems, sick parents, your own health issues—there are so many sources of stress in our modern daily lives. When you experience stress, your body releases powerful chemicals and hormones, including one called cortisol, that prepare your body to fight or flee a perceived threat or danger—the "fight or flight" response. "That response creates a biochemical soup that changes the chemistry of our blood," explains Elissa Epel, PhD, associate professor in the department of psychiatry at the University of California, San Francisco.

The fight or flight response is beneficial in the short run; it helps us deal with a variety of dangerous situations. After the threat has been resolved, hormones level off and your body goes back to baseline. But if these high levels of stress chemicals persist—as they often do when someone is living a high-pressure life—they can be harmful. Instead of protecting the body, they can cause damage to molecules and tissues and lead to a weakened immune system, acne, and other problems, including increased intra-abdominal fat, the kind that puts the body at risk for stroke, heart disease, and high blood pressure. The stress response also triggers higher levels of damaging free radicals, inflammation, and, in some cases, even spikes in insulin and glucose levels that make the body seem prediabetic. And all of these, not surprisingly, can speed up the aging process.

Prolonged stress can also be extremely harmful to the brain. Studies have shown that persistent stress can cause depression and anxiety. It can kill brain cells and damage the hippocampus, the area in charge of memory and learning (research suggests stress actually shrinks this portion of the brain). When damaged, the hippocampus cannot create new memories or access stored ones as efficiently. And because the hippocampus is part of the

Getting a Handle on Stress

In this day and age, it's the rare person who doesn't feel stressed in some way. Rarer still is the person who is managing it well. I say "managing" it because it's really not possible to entirely eliminate stress from your life. But if you organize your life more efficiently and have a few go-to ways to relax, you can significantly lower the wear and tear stress has on your body. Here are a few suggestions for living a lower-stress life.

- List the major sources of stress in your life to identify the big categories.

- Keep a journal for two weeks to identify the more specific triggers. Write down all the situations that make you feel anxious or tense, as well as how you handled (or didn't handle) them. At the end of two weeks, read through your journal. What stressful events can you avoid? Which relationships are making you feel stressed out? Can you improve them, or possibly consider ending them? If you're constantly pressed for time with a day that's way too full, what in your schedule could you possibly eliminate?

- Make sure you are following all the healthy recommendations in this book. Eating healthfully, exercising regularly, and getting enough sleep can go a long way toward helping you cope with stress.

- Have a collection of "emergency stress stoppers" in your arsenal. The American Heart Association recommends these seven ways to calm down.

system that signals the body to stop producing cortisol, levels of the stress hormone can remain out of control and continue to harm the body.

The effects of prolonged stress can even be seen on a cellular level. Epel's research has shown that people with high stress levels have shorter telomeres, which we know is indicative of whole-body aging. (See page 30 for a description of one study involving stress, telomeres, and exercise).

Managing current sources of stress is a must, but it's also important to realize that the stress experienced in the past can play a role in your present-day well-being, too. Research shows that stressful or traumatic life events that you experienced as a child—for instance, losing a parent—can have a powerful and lasting effect. "Really stressful events from childhood can add

1. Count to ten before you speak.
2. Take three to five deep breaths.
3. Walk away from the stressful situation and say you'll handle it later.
4. Go for a walk.
5. Don't be afraid to say "I'm sorry" if you make a mistake.
6. Break down big problems into smaller parts. For example, answer one email or phone call per day instead of dealing with everything at once.
7. Drive in the slow lane or avoid busy roads to help you stay calm while driving.

- Make time for daily relaxation. It's important to determine what helps slow your mind and body down. Maybe it's meditation, yoga, or working out in the gym. It could be reading, sitting down with a cup of tea, listening to music. Find what helps you de-stress and practice it at least once a day.

- Get help if you need it. And I'm not just talking about seeing a therapist, although seeing a therapist can be helpful if you feel that your life is out of control. Consider enrolling in a stress management program at a local hospital, medical center, or community clinic. Someone like a professional organizer or life coach might be able to help you manage your life more efficiently. If you're feeling overwhelmed, talk to your family, friends, colleagues, boss, or even your company's administration. They may be able to help you scale back if you've taken on too many responsibilities.

a couple years to a person's subjective age; they can make people feel older," says Markus Schafer, a sociology researcher at Purdue University. "On the other hand, when people feel in control of their lives and things are going smoothly, they're better able to maintain a sense of youthfulness."

Whether it's stress from the past or stress in the present that you're battling, it may make it more difficult to fight the physical decline that comes with aging. With my own clients, I've seen those overly affected by stress become overwhelmed and have a hard time living up to their eating and exercise goals. When you're stressed out, a comfy couch and a carton of ice cream become a lot more appealing than getting on a treadmill or having a healthy meal—although both of the latter (especially exercise) are good antidotes for stress. Stress also has a tremendous effect on attitude. It can make you feel negative about yourself and your life; it's hard to appreciate all the good things you have when you're overburdened, tense, and pressured. Stress can simply sap all the joy and happiness right out of you.

AGING'S EFFECTS ON THE BODY

There are essentially two ways that we age. The first is called primary aging. "That happens at the cellular level and includes attacks on our cells by free radicals, DNA damage, and the wear and tear on cells, tissues and organs from constant ongoing chemical and other reactions that constitute metabolism," explains Donald Williamson, PhD, an anti-aging researcher and the John Stauffer McIlhenny Professor in Nutrition at Pennington Biomedical Research Center in Louisiana. "Secondary aging is developing a disease such as cancer, atherosclerosis, or diabetes, which can shorten the life span."

Some aspects of aging are obvious. It's apparent, for instance, that the skin changes. Layers within and beneath the skin become thinner, helping to cause sagging and wrinkles—the skin, in a sense, folds in on itself. The skin also becomes less elastic and drier. It grows to be less sensitive to touch, too, and becomes less adept at regulating the body's temperature. Hair loses pigment (the reason we become gray) and hair volume is lost in both men and women.

Body shape can change, too. Most people gain fat, and in many women, fat storage shifts from the hips and thighs to the abdomen. This deep intra-abdominal fat is one of the reasons that the risk of heart disease and diabetes in women dramatically increases after menopause.

One of the more noticeable signs that someone is growing older is the sudden appearance of reading glasses on his or her face. As the lens of the eye becomes less flexible, it makes it harder to focus on objects in the near distance. Vision in dim light also diminishes, and cataracts—clouded lenses—can start forming as early as age forty.

There are also many changes that you can't see, and these changes have an impact on secondary aging. For instance, the thymus, a gland central to the immune system, shrinks, and many of the immune cells decrease in their ability to battle bacteria, viruses, and even cancer cells. The heart muscle degenerates slightly and the valves inside the heart become thicker and stiffer. Arteries are more likely to get clogged with plaque, and blood pressure may increase. The function of most organs declines as well, and cells become less able to divide and reproduce. Some hormone levels rise while others drop, changing the characteristics of many physiological processes such as metabolism and insulin sensitivity. Our sleep architecture—the different stages of sleep—shifts so that we spend less time in deep, refreshing sleep and more time in the lighter phases from which we're more easily awakened.

Significant changes in the muscles, bones, and joints start to occur as well. Muscle fibers shrink and the repair of muscle tissue slows, lowering strength, decreasing the rate at which calories are burned, and making the body more susceptible to obesity. The joints become stiffer and bone mass is lost, increasing the risk of osteoporosis. The vertebrae can also become more compressed, the reason why many people lose height as they grow older.

THE LIGHT AT THE END OF THE TUNNEL

Just reading all of the above, I know, can cause you some despair. No one likes to think of their body (and especially their mind) deteriorating. But there's room for optimism, because you can really make a difference in the rate at which you age and how susceptible you become to age-related diseases. Everything I describe above *can* happen, but it doesn't have to: *How you live can have a significant impact on how your body ages*. In the following chapters, you'll learn about how exercise, good nutrition, skin care, and healthy sleep habits actually change your physiology. Your body will grow chronologically older; there is nothing you can do about that. But you can get physiologically younger. Successful aging isn't an oxymoron. By adhering to the advice in this book, you can substantially lower your likelihood of disease, look and feel younger, and stay strong, vital, sharp, active, and happy. Work at it and you can even turn back the clock twenty years or more—no exaggeration.

Keep Your Health in Check

One of the most important things you can do to fight age-related maladies is to watch for any symptoms of disease. Catching conditions early is key to making a good recovery. Visit your doctor regularly, talk to him or her about any tests that have no set recommendations, and make sure that you are scheduled for the tests that you should have at regular intervals. Here are some guidelines adapted from recommendations from the U.S. Department of Health and Human Services and the American Heart Association. Vaccinations are also very important. Check the Centers for Disease Control and Prevention website (cdc.gov) to see the current recommended vaccinations for your age group.

Screening Tests	Ages 26–39	Ages 40–49	Ages 50–64	Ages 65 and older
Full check-up, including weight and height	Discuss with your physician.			
Thyroid (TSH) test	Discuss with your physician.			
Blood pressure test	At least every 2 years.			
Cholesterol test	Every 5 years; more frequently if your cholesterol is over 200 or you are a man over 45 or a woman over 50.			
Bone density screen		Discuss with your physician.		Get a bone mineral density test at least once. Talk to your physician about repeat testing.
Diabetes: Blood glucose or A1c test	Discuss with your physician.	Start at age 45, then every 3 years.	Every 3 years.	
Chlamydia test	Get this test if you have new or multiple partners.			
Sexually transmitted infection (STI) tests	Both partners should get tested for STIs, including HIV, before initiating sexual intercourse.			
Colorectal health (use 1 of these 3 methods): Fecal occult blood test			Yearly.	Yearly. Older than age 75, discuss with your physician.

Screening Tests	Ages 26–39	Ages 40–49	Ages 50–64	Ages 65 and older
Flexible sigmoidoscopy (with fecal occult blood test)			Every 5 years.	Every 5 years. Older than age 75, discuss with your physician.
Colonoscopy			Every 10 years.	Every 10 years. Older than age 75, discuss with your doctor or nurse.
Comprehensive eye exam	Discuss with your physician.	Get a baseline exam at age 40, then every 2–4 years or as your doctor advises.	Every 2–4 years until age 55, then every 1–3 years until age 65, or as your doctor advises.	Every 1–2 years.
Hearing test	Starting at age 18, then every 10 years.	Every 10 years.	Every 3 years.	
Mole exam	Monthly mole self-exam; by a physician as part of a routine full checkup.			
For Women Only:				
Mammogram		Every 1–2 years. Discuss with your physician.		
Clinical breast exam	At least every 3 years.	Yearly.		
Pap test	Every 2 years. Women 30 and older, every 3 years.	Every 3 years.		
Pelvic exam	Yearly.			
For Men Only:				
Digital rectal exam		Discuss with your physician.		
Prostate-specific antigen test (PSA)		Discuss with your physician.		
Testicular exam	Discuss with your physician.			

CHAPTER 2

The Ultimate Anti-Aging Weapon: Exercise

A FEW YEARS AGO I was waiting to board a plane when I noticed the man standing next to me, a guy who appeared to be in his late sixties, wearing a really cool pair of glasses. I complimented him on the glasses, and just as he was telling me they were a gift from his daughter, I glanced down at his boarding pass and saw the name "LaLanne." I immediately thought back to how, growing up, I had watched my mom exercise along to Jack LaLanne's TV show. I'm surprised I didn't recognize him right away, but once I realized who he was I knew that he couldn't be in his sixties. When I got home I looked it up and confirmed it: Jack LaLanne was in his early *nineties*.

As a champion of combining cardiovascular exercise and strength training for good health and fitness, LaLanne was way ahead of his time. And it obviously paid off. The man I met that day in the airport not only looked way younger than his years, but he was strong and healthy and had a youthful way about him. If there ever was an advertisement for the anti-aging benefits of exercise, I was looking at it right there. When it comes to reversing the aging process, nothing touches exercise.

If you think about it, it makes complete sense. Aging, as I described in the previous chapter, is by its very definition the loss and breakdown of tissues within the body. Physical activity, to the contrary, builds up tissues within the body. That's obvious when you look at the musculature of devoted exercisers, but exercise also builds up tissue and enhances cellular activity in ways that you can't even see. For instance, think about what exercise does for the body in terms of disease prevention. Studies show that the risk of obesity, heart disease, hypertension, stroke, diabetes, cancer, and just about every other condition that leads to disability and/or early death goes up with age. But people who exercise regularly defy those statistics. They stay leaner and have more robust cardiovascular systems, better insulin sensitivity, and stronger immune systems. Daily physical activity sends a message to your brain and your body to stay young and vibrant, and as a result exercisers typically live not only longer but higher-quality lives.

By "higher quality" I mean that exercisers don't suffer the same physical and psychological decline that sedentary people usually do—a decline that often begins as early as age twenty-five. When people *don't* exercise, they experience both muscle and bone loss, setting themselves up for weakness and the risk of injury in their older years. Exercisers, on the other hand, maintain strong muscles and bones, allowing them to continue leading active, on-the-go lives. Research also suggests that older exercisers have sharper memories and cognitive skills, and that they're more optimistic and satisfied with life. Because exercise helps ease depression and anxiety, people who exercise regularly tend to be calmer, too. That alone is useful in the fight against aging, since we know that stress contributes to the deterioration of the body. Recently, a study at the University of California, San Francisco, found that women with a lot of stress in their lives who were physically active had longer telomeres than stressed women who were sedentary. (Longer telomeres, as you might remember from chapter 1, are a mark of younger, healthier cells.) Exercise, we now know, has benefits right down to the molecular level.

It even affects how other people perceive you. When English researchers quizzed people on their perceptions of sixty-five-year-old exercisers versus non-exercisers of the same age, they judged the exercisers to be friendlier, more hardworking, kinder, happier, more sociable, and better-looking than the non-exercisers. And here's the kicker: The people making the judgments were basing their perceptions on a written statement that mentioned who exercised and who did not but included very little physical description; they had never even *seen* the sixty-five-year-olds.

A FOUNDATION FOR LIVING LIFE TO THE FULLEST

A friend of mine loves to tell the story of her grandfather, a man who was active all his life and regularly played softball until he was ninety-three. One night, her grandfather was visiting the family when a knock sounded on the door. It was the next-door neighbor, who'd seen a prowler on the side of my friend's family's house. My friend's grandfather, in his early eighties at the time, ran to the side of the house, shouted out at the prowler — a young man — then took off running after him down the alley. A few blocks later her grandfather caught the man (he let him go with a warning), and his feat went down in family history.

Hopefully, you'll never have to demonstrate your physical proficiency in such a dramatic way, but I tell the story to remind you that the benefits of being physically fit go well beyond obtaining a lean, toned, and younger-looking body. The most important thing exercise does for you is keep you living an active and independent life. Being able to walk quickly when you're late and climb the stairs of a stadium at a ball game without your heart racing. Having the strength to pull your luggage off the baggage carousel at the airport and the agility to set up a tent. Possessing the stamina to hike the Grand Canyon and the power to cycle through vineyards. Having the flexibility to swing a tennis racquet and the energy to swim in the ocean and walk on the sand. Even if these types of things are no problem for you now, they very well could be if you don't take preventive measures.

As I frequently say, we were meant to move. And yet, as a society, we barely do. We text, we email, we push remote control and elevator buttons, we step onto escalators, we put dishes in the dishwasher, we drive, and we sit, sit, sit. According to an American Cancer Society study, women who are otherwise inactive and sit six hours a day increase their likelihood of early death by 98 percent compared to women who are very active and sit less than three hours per day. That's astounding! We've become very apathetic about moving our bodies and we're paying the price in runaway rates of obesity and diabetes.

The Aging Brain on Exercise

Arthur F. Kramer is what you might call the sage of the aging brain and exercise. The director of the Beckman Institute of Advanced Science and professor in the Department of Psychology and Neuroscience at the University of Illinois at Urbana, he has led numerous studies looking at what happens to the brains of older people when they exercise. His work makes a strong case for working out to stay mentally sharp as well as for picking up exercise no matter what your age. "We know from our studies that you can take older people who are almost professional couch potatoes and have them start exercising late in life and get pretty dramatic benefits," says Kramer. "Studies also show that exercise improves cognitive function in people with Parkinson's disease, multiple sclerosis, and Alzheimer's."

In Kramer and his colleagues' most recent study, they invited sixty-five of those professional couch potatoes, ages fifty-nine to eighty, to join a walking group for a year. At the end of the year, the researchers looked at the walkers' brains with high-resolution imaging and found that they had increased brain connectivity and improved scores on cognitive tests. Connectivity, which means that different parts of the brain are acting in sync, typically declines with age, and so does cognition. By contrast, a control group in Kramer's study that did only stretching exercises had no improvement in either cognition or connectivity.

Other work coauthored by Kramer has found that older people who started with fifteen minutes of walking and built up to forty-five minutes showed increases in brain volume in areas that usually show significant age-related deterioration. The volunteers in that study ranged in age from sixty through seventy-nine. "There may be a point of no return when you're too old for exercise to improve your brain function," says Kramer. "But so far we haven't found it."

For every step forward we've taken in technology, we've taken a step back in regard to our health. But there's a remedy for that: a solid, well-rounded exercise program that compensates for the loss of activity in the way we live our lives today. That's a good description of the anti-aging fitness plan waiting for you at the end of this chapter. It's designed expressly to counterbalance the way modern life facilitates and even accelerates the aging process. You may be surprised at how much exercise I'm going to ask you to do; I'm probably going to tell you to move more than you initially want to. But engaging in structured exercise every day is how you fight back against aging. You can't just go for a quick walk around the block on your lunch hour and expect to get all the anti-aging benefits I mentioned. It takes more time and more energy—it takes a solid investment in yourself—but it's well worth it. The rewards are life-changing, and if you develop a strong exercise habit, they'll stay with you for a lifetime.

It's no accident that the exercise chapter is here in the front of this book. A comprehensive exercise regimen is the foundation of any anti-aging program; its contributions to overall youthfulness and well-being are unparalleled. Not only is regular physical activity transformative on its own, but it also acts as a gateway to improvement in all the other areas we touch on in this book. People who are physically active tend to eat more healthfully. They have good circulation so their skin gets the oxygen and nutrients it needs to look—and act—younger. Exercisers sleep better, too, staying longer in the more rejuvenating stage of slumber. They also typically cope better with stress and often have a more positive outlook on life. Exercise directly or indirectly relates to everything else you can do to turn back the clock.

HOW EXERCISE SLOWS THE AGING PROCESS

If you've been physically active all your life, you're probably already "physiologically" younger than your chronological age. But if you're a lapsed exerciser or really haven't ever done much physical activity at all, you can still make significant headway in the fight against aging. Though I wouldn't go as far as to say that exercise is the fountain of youth, evidence suggests that, in many ways, it's the closest thing we've got. Here are some reasons why:

Exercise prevents the deterioration of muscle and bone. By some calculations, most women begin losing about 1 percent of muscle mass per year after the age of forty; men begin losing muscle in their *twenties*. That loss of muscle tissue also contributes to a big loss in strength: Muscular strength can drop by as much as 30 to 40 percent by the time you're in your eighties.

A lot of people are resigned to their musculature growing flabbier and weaker with age; they figure it's a fact of life. But the truth is, it's not inevitable. The blame for most muscle tissue and muscle strength loss can be laid squarely at the feet of inactivity. I hate to trot out an old cliché, but it's undeniably true: Use it or lose it. Countless studies have shown that if you strength train you can regain and/or maintain muscle volume, endurance, and power — even if you're ninety years old.

Beyond the obvious — no one wants to end up as the older person (or even the middle-aged person) who has trouble pushing open a door or transporting his body around — there are good reasons to preserve muscle. Muscle tissue is calorie-hungry, meaning that it takes a lot of energy to maintain it. The more muscle you have, the more calories you burn each day, which helps you limit weight gain. One reason that so many people end up gaining weight in middle age — and having a higher likelihood of obesity-related conditions such as heart disease, high blood pressure, and diabetes — is because muscle loss has left them with a lowered ability to burn calories. When you hold on to muscle, you hold on to your calorie-burning power, too.

Strength training is the best way to build and preserve muscle. When you strength train by doing exercises with dumbbells (my preference for most people), resistance bands, or weight machines, the load creates microtears in the muscles, and the body, in repairing those tears, generates larger, denser muscles. Another thing strength training does is activate nerves within the muscles that allow them to respond to challenges more effectively.

Strength training also allows you to take aim at another common age-related issue: bone loss. Bone tissue may seem static, but in fact your body is constantly breaking down bone and rebuilding it. When you're young, your body breaks down and rebuilds bone in equal measure, but the balance gradually shifts as you get older. By the time most people are in their forties and fifties, a confluence of factors, including, in women, loss of estrogen, has created enough of an imbalance to cause bone thinning. People who have a particularly large imbalance of breakdown and buildup are at risk for the brittle bone disease osteoporosis. But when you strength train, your muscles tug on your bones, triggering the rebuilding process and keeping the bones healthy. Weight-bearing cardiovascular exercise — anything that involves impact, such as running, walking, stair stepping, aerobic dance — also helps build bone. It's worth noting that when you strength train *and* choose a weight-bearing activity as your cardiovascular exercise, you double your efforts to prevent age-related bone loss.

Exercise keeps age-related diseases at bay and reduces the likelihood of middle-age spread. Cardiovascular exercise (also known as aerobic exercise) has different anti-aging effects than strength training, but they are no less amazing. I'll get to the specifics about those effects shortly, but first let me explain what it means to improve your cardiovascular system, which is made up of your heart and the network of blood vessels that course through your body. When your cardiovascular system is fit, it has a heightened ability to process oxygen and deliver it to your working muscles. That makes movement, especially sustained movement, noticeably easier. Running to catch a bus, going up stairs, walking to the store, keeping up with a child, require far less effort when you have cardiovascular power and endurance. A fit cardiovascular system even works more efficiently when you're at rest. With all that energy saved you inevitably feel less fatigued.

Physical activities that accelerate your breathing and make your heart work harder for a continuous and extended period of time significantly improve your cardiovascular system. These type of workouts all involve repetitive motion and engage your large muscle groups, but most important they allow you to sustain movement. Brisk walking, running, swimming, cycling, elliptical training, stair stepping, and aerobic dance all fit the bill. By contrast, an activity such as tennis, which is great for balance and hand-eye coordination, isn't an ideal cardiovascular activity, because it typically requires too much starting and stopping. Strength training is another activity that is sometimes thought to have aerobic benefits; however, while it's wonderful for muscle strengthening, it doesn't challenge the cardiovascular system.

Though you're born with an innate amount of cardiovascular ability (or aerobic capacity, as it's often called), it can begin to decline at a relatively early age. If you're very inactive, the deterioration starts sometime in your twenties and then accelerates with each decade. But if you engage in consistent, moderate-to-high-level cardiovascular exercise, you can maintain your cardiovascular ability and even see improvement well into your thirties, forties, and beyond. Regular cardiovascular exercise also causes other changes in the body that significantly lower the risk of many age-related diseases. For instance, it's long been known that cardiovascular exercise raises levels of HDL (good) cholesterol, helping to protect against heart disease. It also increases insulin sensitivity, lowering the risk of diabetes, and reduces inflammation, which is linked to a number of life-threatening conditions (see box on page 37).

Like strength training, cardiovascular exercise helps you fight midlife weight gain, too. It's believed that most adults gain about ten pounds per decade, but data collected for the National Runners' Health Study, a project being conducted at the U.S. Department of Energy's Lawrence Berkeley National Laboratory in California, shows that people who are consistently active put on significantly fewer pounds than that. And most likely it's not just because exercise burns calories while you're doing it. When you regularly engage in cardiovascular exercise, you increase the production and storage of something called aerobic enzymes. These enzymes do a great job of boosting your metabolism, the rate at which you burn calories, as well as helping the body burn more fat. In large part due to these enzymes, regular exercisers simply incinerate more calories twenty-four hours a day. Since the metabolism typically slows down with age, that's a boost everyone over the age of thirty can use.

There's another way cardiovascular exercise affects body weight. Men are prone to gaining weight in their bellies all through their lives. As women get older, that tendency increases and asserts itself in them as well. Most women typically gain fat in their arms, legs, and hips until menopause, when hormone levels shift and they begin storing what is known as intra-abdominal fat, located deep in the abdominal cavity. This fat puts you at greater risk for heart disease, stroke, and cancer. Remarkably, cardiovascular exercise seems to target intra-abdominal fat. One study found that women

Offsetting the Aging of the Immune System

Whenever there's an outbreak of a flu virus or food poisoning, the elderly are among those who get hit the hardest. One reason that's likely is that the immune system's ability to fight off infection tends to decline with age. That said, several studies have found that physically active elderly people have greater immune cell function than elderly people who don't move around much. We also know that moderate exercise increases activity of natural killer cells (a type of immune cell that can destroy tumor and other harmful cells) in people of all ages, undoubtedly the reason regular exercisers get fewer colds and flu and miss significantly fewer days of work. Natural killer cells also appear to help wipe out cancer cells, another way they keep you safe.

While it may be too early to say that exercise stops the natural aging of the immune system, researchers at McMaster University in Ontario, Canada, found that it seems to produce changes in the body that compensate for age-related reductions in antibodies. One of those changes is a lower level of inflammation. Inflammation has an important role in the body; when triggered by some kind of injury or infection, it helps the body heal by promoting more immune activity in the affected area. But chronic, low-grade inflammation actually worsens unhealthful conditions, doing more harm than good, and it's been implicated as a culprit in numerous conditions, including heart disease, cancer, Parkinson's disease, Alzheimer's disease, and autoimmune diseases such as rheumatoid arthritis and lupus. There is also some evidence to suggest that chronic inflammation — which can be a side effect of obesity, among other things — can lead to DNA mutations and, ultimately, the development of cancer.

There are a few different ways that exercise may reduce inflammation. One is by lowering levels of an inflammatory protein called C-reactive protein (CRP). CRP levels in the body increase with age, one reason we become more prone to developing inflammation-related diseases as we get older. Exercise reduces the levels of proteins called pro-inflammatory cytokines and increases levels of an *anti*-inflammatory form of cytokines. In a roundabout way, exercise may also rid the body of inflammation by decreasing body fat: Body fat actually produces pro-inflammatory cytokines that cause inflammation.

on an aerobic exercise program lost 3 to 7 percent of their belly fat — without even changing their eating habits.

Exercise changes the body at the cellular level. Many of the anti-aging benefits of exercise don't necessarily show up on cholesterol tests or on the scale, but they're significant nonetheless. One of the most exciting areas of anti-aging research is the attempt to discover how exercise affects the life span and function of cells. For instance, researchers at the University of Colorado at Boulder recently compared the white blood cells of people aged fifty-five to seventy-two who did regular aerobic exercise to those of both their sedentary peers and younger people aged eighteen to thirty-two who exercised regularly. What they found was that the older exercisers had longer telomeres than the older sedentary folks, and their telomeres were not significantly different from those of younger exercisers. "Two general 'anti-aging' strategies would be either to decrease the rate of telomere shortening, or to increase the rate of telomere repair so that they maintain their length," says Thomas LaRocca, a PhD candidate and lead author of the study. "Aerobic exercise may stimulate pathways and enzymes in the body that do both."

There's also evidence that regular cardiovascular exercise positively affects mitochondria, little factories in the cells that manufacture ATP, the main source of energy driving just about every biological process in the body. Mitochondrial function is known to decline with age. However, work by researchers at the Mayo Clinic College of Medicine has shown that older people who regularly engage in cardiovascular exercise have better mitochondrial functioning and capacity than young people who don't exercise.

One of the ways that the mitochondria play a role in aging is by providing energy to replace damaged proteins, thereby preventing the deterioration of many tissues and structures in the body. K. Sreekumaran Nair, MD, PhD, an endocrinologist and an author of the Mayo Clinic study, gives this example: "One reason you lose strength with age is that the proteins that enable the muscles to contract become damaged; it's not only due to loss of muscle tissue," he says. "With better mitochondrial function, you can synthesize new contractile proteins." Nair and his colleagues also found that cardiovascular exercise increases the expression of SIRT3, which is sometimes called the longevity gene. SIRT3 is one of a number of enzymes called sirtuins that make cells less susceptible to an early death. Calorie restriction and the compound resveratrol (which you can read more about in chapter 3) also increase production of SIRT3.

WHAT IS FITNESS?

I've just told you many of the ways that strengthening your muscles and training your cardiovascular system can improve and even extend your life. But I don't want to give you the idea that attaining muscular strength or cardiovascular endurance or both is all there is to being fit. Fitness actually has many qualities, and each of them needs to be addressed by a comprehensive fitness program.

If I asked you to think of someone who's the epitome of fitness, you might visualize an elite athlete such as a marathon runner. After all, what could be more representative of fitness than the ability to run twenty-six miles? But marathon runners are often like other exercisers who stick to one sport and think of themselves as fit yet are wanting in other areas. That marathon runner, for instance, while definitely possessed of excellent cardiovascular fitness, might throw her back out bending down to pick up her briefcase. She may lack core strength and flexibility. Think, too, of the guy at the gym who can bench 350 pounds but can't run up the stairs of the subway without panting. He has limited cardiovascular endurance.

Whereas a high level of cardiovascular fitness and muscle strength will help you reap the anti-aging rewards I've talked about, to be truly "fit" you also need to be proficient in ways that allow you to function at a high level as you go about your daily life. You don't just want to be good at a particular type of exercise; you want to be good at all aspects of fitness, allowing you to be good at life. What's more, you want to be fit in ways that will keep you from getting injured so that you can consistently participate in cardiovascular and muscle-strengthening exercise and at a level that will maximize all the anti-aging benefits I cited.

Cardiovascular endurance and muscular strength are critical aspects of fitness, but there are six other important qualities of overall fitness that I haven't mentioned yet. These qualities also tend to weaken with age if you don't address them. The first is flexibility, the ability of your muscles to give and allow your joints a good range of motion. Flexibility enables your body to move freely and comfortably, but as the muscles shorten and stiffen with age, flexibility wanes, restricting movement. Abdominal and back ("core") strength is critical too, because it protects your spine from wear and tear and stabilizes the entire body when you lift, push, or pull anything. Core strength also improves your posture, keeping your body upright so it doesn't succumb to hunching from computer use or general fatigue. Strengthening key stabilizing muscles is also important. When well conditioned, certain muscles protect other areas of the body. Strengthening the calves, for instance, helps prevent shin splints; strengthening the muscles around the shoulder girdle helps prevent rotator cuff tears.

Agility, the ability to quickly change direction and react to changing circumstances, is another important area of fitness, as is balance, being able to control and maintain your body's position. Last but not least is hand-eye coordination, the ability to assess the location and/or size of an object and quickly initiate the appropriate muscular response in your hands — or even your feet or other parts of your body (it should really be called body-eye coordination). It helps keep you safe in everyday ways by, for instance, allowing you to quickly sidestep a rock on the sidewalk and drive a car proficiently. It also makes you better at engaging in recreational activities such as golf, bowling, Frisbee, pool, Ping-Pong, and racquetball (in fact, practicing these activities helps you maintain hand-eye coordination).

This might sound overwhelming — it's a lot to cover — but rest assured that you don't need separate workouts to get fit in all of these areas. There's a lot of overlap, and many exercises cover several aspects of fitness. The comprehensive plan beginning on page 48 is going to help you cover all your bases in a methodical and economical way. Think of it this way: Your goal should be to establish a basic level of fitness — it's commonly called functional fitness — that includes all the elements I just listed as well as moderate amounts of cardiovascular endurance and all-over muscular strength and endurance. Together these elements will allow you to comfortably walk up stairs, bend down to pick things up, reach for a box on a high shelf without straining a muscle, be quick and coordinated enough to catch a dish that's slipped out of your hands, and rapidly sidestep an obstacle in your path without twisting an ankle. They also help you get out and do fun things and perform them at higher levels: skiing or snowshoeing in the mountains, sightseeing in big cities, cycling on a long bike path, hiking in the hills, canoeing on a lake. It's easier and more enjoyable to do just about any activity when you're in possession of overall fitness.

Let's go back to my initial question, What does it mean to be fit? Being fit means all of the areas of your body are functioning well; you've trained and optimized all the qualities of fitness. You can tell when someone is fit because he or she is able not only to get through the day comfortably and safely, but also to participate in many activities at a higher level and without injury.

You can attain this baseline level of functional fitness — and many anti-aging benefits — by training at Level I in the *20 Years Younger* exercise plan. The plan also allows you to progress and achieve even greater levels of cardiovascular endurance and muscular strength (which will ramp up the anti-aging payoff). I think just about everyone who is willing to commit to fitness can rise to Level II. It's more demanding, but doable — and the benefits are that much greater. Level III is very challenging. I realize that not everyone is going to be able to fit Level III into his or her life; it's a lot of exercise. But it's also the ultimate comprehensive anti-aging program. If inspiration strikes, and I hope that it will, you will be well rewarded for your efforts.

THE *20 YEARS YOUNGER* ANTI-AGING EXERCISE PLAN

There are three things that make this exercise plan different from other types of fitness programs. One is that it emphasizes variety so that you hit all the areas of fitness essential to halting the aging process: flexibility, core strength, stabilization, agility, balance and hand-eye coordination, cardiovascular endurance, and muscle strength. Most exercise programs tend to have a narrower target. An exercise plan for weight loss, for instance, might have you focusing primarily on calorie burning—but at the expense of other aspects of your physiology that are also affected by age. By contrast, this program doesn't have you chewing up a lot of time trying to reach a limited goal; instead, it casts a wide net that lets you turn back the clock in virtually *all* areas of fitness relating to aging.

The second important thing about this plan is that although it requires a fairly substantial commitment on your part, I'm only asking you to take on as much as you can handle at a time. There are three levels and you can choose just how far you want to go. If you haven't been doing much physical activity lately (or any at all), start at Level I, which primarily focuses on functional conditioning and helping you establish a base of cardiovascular endurance and muscular strength. In a matter of weeks, you'll feel stronger and notice that you get through your day with less effort. You should also notice that you're sleeping better and your skin looks more vibrant. Having laid the groundwork at Level I, you can progress to Level II. (If you're already a regular exerciser, you can probably skip the beginning level and jump right into Level II.) Here I ratchet up the challenge, asking you to spend more time on cardiovascular exercise and muscle strengthening. The payoff is considerable: This level of exercise can bring about substantial changes in body fat, the strength of your muscles, the fitness of your heart, and your mood—changes that will not only benefit your health but help push back the clock to a greater degree.

I have had clients who started an exercise program reluctantly, committing to do "something" only because their doctor warned them that they had better get active or face the music. To their surprise, many of these initially reluctant exercisers get inspired not only to take it to the next level but, in a manner of speaking, to shoot for the stars. They run marathons, enter triathlons, or simply make physical activity among their highest priorities. This is what I'm hoping will happen with you. Once you reap the rewards of Level II, you may be inspired to invest additional time and energy to move up to

Level III. I want to stress that *all* levels of the plan have anti-aging benefits, but the advanced level does the most to help you maintain muscle and bone, fight middle-age spread, and lower your risk of disease. It's the best opportunity you have to recapture (and maybe even improve upon!) your youth.

The third thing that makes this program different is that it includes what I call lifetime sports and recreational activities. Activities such as golf, tennis, and bowling help you stay active during your leisure time; most important for our anti-aging purposes, many of them also help you work on agility, balance, and hand-eye coordination. Another reason I recommend them is that many of them are social activities, too, and we know that keeping socially active is a powerful predictor of longevity.

Before I give you the specifics of the comprehensive plan, let's go over some basics for each of the components.

Cardiovascular Exercise

Most people find a type of cardiovascular exercise they like and stick with it, sometimes even doing the same type of exercise every day. I'm going to encourage you to take a different approach and choose not one type of aerobic exercise, but two, even three. This is referred to as cross training. Each type of exercise works your body in a different way, so when you expand your repertoire, you expand the number of muscles trained and the number of ways you can fight aging. In addition, when your schedule includes variety, you lower your risk of developing an overuse injury that will sideline you and keep you from doing any exercise at all. Having more than one go-to workout also keeps your week more interesting.

You can also avoid burnout and maximize the benefits you get by shaking up your workout routine every six months. I'll give you an example. Say you walk on Monday, Tuesday, Wednesday, and Friday and ride your bike on Thursday and Saturday. After six months you might switch—cycle four days a week and walk on two—or replace cycling with the elliptical trainer. Though you need to spend adequate amounts of time establishing a base level of fitness in each type of activity, once you have that base (and six months is enough to let you establish it), you can change things around without losing the activity-specific conditioning you've gained.

When you go about deciding which aerobic workouts to choose, consider that some do a better job of improving your cardiovascular system than others. Of course, I think you should select the ones that give you the biggest payoffs for your effort, but it's also important to choose something you like; otherwise, you're not going to stay motivated for long.

Use the roundup on page 53 to guide you. It tells you the pros and cons of each type of workout and gives you my opinion on how effective they are for achieving your aerobic and anti-aging goals. Even if you think you know everything about every type of aerobic exercise, give it a read. Some of the particulars might surprise you.

How long, how often, and how hard do you need to do cardiovascular exercise? On the exercise plan chart I'll give you a specific number of minutes you should accomplish each week. Ideally, every workout should be at least twenty continuous minutes; however, you can choose how to break up the rest of the minutes. You can also choose what days of the week you want to engage in cardiovascular exercise, but don't take off two days in a row. To determine the proper intensity of your exercise, I'm going to introduce you to the Perceived Exertion Scale on page 58. This tool helps you gauge how exercise feels on a scale of 0 to 10 primarily using your breathing as a guide. To get maximum cardiovascular benefits, you'll need to work out at a 7 or 8 on the scale. Not working hard enough (below level 7 or 8 on the Perceived Exertion Scale) is the number one reason people don't see the results they want.

If you aren't very fit, it will take very little movement to get your heart and breathing rates up into the range they need to be in. For instance, a slower walking speed of 3.5 miles per hour may be enough to get a beginner up to an 8 on the Perceived Exertion Scale, but a relatively fit walker may need to walk at a speed of 5 miles per hour (or faster) to get into that range or walk up a significant grade. The point is, no one can tell you what numbers to punch into the treadmill control panel to get *your* best individual cardiovascular workout. Listening to your body will tell you if you're working hard enough. Be sure to learn the Perceived Exertion Scale.

Counting Steps Per Day

The number of steps you take per day, whether you're formally going for a walk or just moving around as you do your daily activities, counts toward improving your fitness in Level I, but only Level I. That's because although it helps you attain a good functional level of fitness, it's typically not vigorous enough to help you achieve higher levels of fitness. To determine your number of steps per day, you'll need a pedometer, a clip-on counting device that you can wear all day. You can purchase one at most sporting goods stores or on www.20YearsYounger.com.

Strength Training

If you haven't ever lifted weights before, the process can seem daunting. But strength training is not difficult to master, and it takes very little time to complete an entire program when it's done properly. Level I starts with six basic strength-training exercises; if you decide to go all the way up to Level III, there are quite a few more. Most of the exercises call for dumbbells; however, they also can be done on the type of weight machines you typically find in a gym. A few of the exercises in Level III are only done on weight machines.

There is always some question as to whether it's best to use heavy weights and fewer repetitions (the number of times you raise and lower a weight or push against or pull a weight machine) or lighter weights and more repetitions. For anti-aging purposes in particular, I recommend relatively heavy weights and fewer reps — eight to ten unless otherwise noted — which is the best way to build strength and maintain muscle. Lighter weights and more repetitions can do a good job of toning muscles and improving muscular endurance; however, you'll already be enhancing both those qualities with cardiovascular exercise. Repetitions are organized into sets. It's possible to get some good benefits from one set, and it's a current trend to recommend only one. But for the maximum anti-aging payoff, I'd like you to gradually work up to three sets per exercise. In between sets, rest only fifteen to thirty seconds (the closer to the lower end of that range you can go, the better). Fatigue is what prompts the changes in your muscles' anatomy, and too much rest lessens the strength-building effect. It's also important to breathe properly as you strength train. Always breathe out during the exertion phase and in as you're returning to starting position. For instance, when you're doing a biceps curl, you breathe out as you curl the weights up toward your shoulders and in as you lower them back down.

Strength is very individual, so it's necessary to go through a little trial and error to determine how many pounds you should be lifting for each exercise. Here's the method I like to use. To select the proper weight, start with very light resistance, then go up to the next weight, then the next, until you find a weight that is heavy enough to make your muscles feel fatigued after lifting it eight to ten times. By fatigued I mean that it's difficult to accomplish the last repetition. (If you feel *slightly* sore the next day or two after training, it's a sign that the weights were right.) If the weights are heavy enough, you may only be able to do eight reps during a second set and even fewer during a third set. If you can easily do ten reps on the third set, your weights are probably too light.

As you get stronger, you'll need to increase the weight you lift. If it becomes too easy, then you're not going to get all the benefits you could be getting. I also recommend mixing up your workouts when you can. Strength-training exercises can get a little stale after a while, and your body will respond better to the challenge if you weave in alternative exercises every six to eight months. There are, for instance, several different types of biceps exercises. If you usually do traditional biceps curls, you might try something like pull-ups (or modified pull-ups) instead. When I go on vacation, I often use weight machines in the hotel gym that are different from the ones I use at home. You'll find alternatives for all of the strength-training exercises on page 70.

Stretches and Core Exercises

There are nine stretches and core exercises in Level I of the plan, eleven in Level II, and thirteen in Level III. Though that sounds like a lot, they actually take relatively little time to perform. I recommend that you do them every day. On days that you're doing other exercise, the best time to do these exercises is *after* your cardiovascular or strength-training workout. You want to stretch when your muscles are warm and blood flow makes them more elastic; stretching cold muscles can cause injury. If you're not doing a sweat-inducing workout that day, at least take a short walk or do something to heat up your body a bit before you stretch. In most cases, it's best to hold a stretch for fifteen to thirty seconds and repeat two to three times. Bouncing is a bad idea, and another way to set yourself up for injury. You don't have to limit your stretching to just these few exercises. Gently stretch your body at intervals throughout the day (again, make sure you're body is warm first), and consider taking yoga or Pilates classes to achieve even greater strength and flexibility.

Generally fifteen repetitions for each core exercise works well. Contrary to popular belief, you don't need to do crunches all day long to get good results. I'll have you start with one set of each exercise then work up to two, then on to three.

Lifetime Sports and Recreational Activities

The reason I refer to these as "lifetime" activities is because you should be able to do them at any age. They all hit one or more of three important qualities of fitness: agility, balance, and hand eye coordination. Get in the habit of participating in them now and you'll always have a way to stay vibrant and active. Many of the activities on the list on pages 78–79 are things you can do with family, friends, or a significant other. Use the opportunity to get the people you care about doing something beneficial for their health, too. And reap the anti-aging benefits of spending time with others (read more about social interaction and aging in chapter 6).

In the list I note which of these activities help you improve balance and hand-eye coordination in particular. If you choose a recreational activity that doesn't provide very much balance conditioning, I recommend that you try performing your strength-training exercises while on a balance apparatus such as the BOSU ball. Keep in mind, too, that some of the lifetime sports can double as your cardiovascular exercise. Skiing (cross-country or downhill), kayaking, walking, swimming, skating — anything that allows for sustained movement and a high oxygen consumption will work.

THE PROGRAM

Level I

CARDIOVASCULAR EXERCISE

Choose activities from the list on page 53.

A minimum of 200 minutes/week — break up as you like; never two days off in a row.

Alternative for beginners: 70,000 steps/week — count steps every day (see page 45).

STRENGTH TRAINING

Start with one set; work up to two sets by month two; work up to three sets by month three. Eight to ten repetitions per set. Three days/week.

1. Heel Raise

2. Shrug Roll

3. Squat

4. Chest Press

5. Biceps Curl

6. Thumbs Down

STRETCHES

Perform each stretch two to three times every day.

1. Hamstring Stretch

2. Quadriceps Stretch

3. Upper Calf Stretch

4. Lower Calf Stretch

5. Middle and Lower Back Stretch

CORE EXERCISES

Start with one set; work up to two sets by month two. Fifteen repetitions per set. Do every day.

1. Basic Crunch

2. Upper Abdominal Crunch

3. Twisting Trunk Curl Crunch

4. Alternating Arm and Leg Raise

LIFETIME SPORTS AND RECREATION

Choose from the list on page 79 — a minimum of one time/week.

If you *don't* choose an activity that covers both balance and hand-eye coordination, do your strength-training exercises on a balancing apparatus.

Level II

CARDIOVASCULAR EXERCISE

A minimum of 300 minutes/week — break up as you like; never two days off in a row.

STRENGTH TRAINING

Three days/week; three sets; eight to ten repetitions/set.

1. Heel Raise

2. Shrug Roll

3. Squat

4. Chest Press

5. Biceps Curl

6. Thumbs Down

7. Lunge

8. One-Arm Row

9. Dumbbell Fly

10. Triceps Extension

11. Shoulder Press

12. External Rotation

STRETCHES

Perform each stretch two to three times every day.

1. Hamstring Stretch

2. Quadriceps Stretch

3. Upper Calf Stretch

4. Lower Calf Stretch

5. Middle and Lower Back Stretch

CORE EXERCISES

Two sets; fifteen repetitions/set. Do every day.

1. Basic Crunch

2. Upper Abdominal Crunch

3. Twisting Trunk Curl Crunch

4. Alternating Arm and Leg Raise

5. Extended Arm Crunch

6. Vertical Leg Crunch

LIFETIME SPORTS AND RECREATION

A minimum of two times/week.

Level III

CARDIOVASCULAR EXERCISE

400 minutes/week — break up as you like; never two days off in a row.

STRENGTH TRAINING

Three days/week; three sets; eight to ten repetitions per set. This list is long, so if time is short you may want to divide it up and do half the exercises one day, the other half the next, with one day off. It won't technically be three times a week, but it is still an effective way to accomplish your goals.

1. Heel Raise

2. Shrug Roll

3. Squat

4. Chest Press

5. Biceps Curl

6. Thumbs Down

7. Lunge

8. One-Arm Row

9. Dumbbell Fly

10. Triceps Extension

11. Shoulder Press

12. External Rotation

13. Leg Extension

14. Leg Curl

15. Lateral Raise

16. Upright Row

17. Incline Chest Press

18. Frontal Raise

19. Lat Pull-Down

STRETCHES

Perform each stretch two to three times every day.

1. Hamstring Stretch

2. Quadriceps Stretch

3. Upper Calf Stretch

4. Lower Calf Stretch

5. Middle and Lower Back Stretch

CORE EXERCISES

Two sets; fifteen repetitions/set. Do every day.

1. Basic Crunch

2. Upper Abdominal Crunch

3. Twisting Trunk Curl Crunch

4. Alternating Arm and Leg Raise

5. Extended Arm Crunch

6. Vertical Leg Crunch

7. Reverse Trunk Curl

8. Incline Sit-Up

LIFETIME SPORTS AND RECREATION

A minimum of two times/week.

CARDIOVASCULAR WORKOUTS

All aerobic workouts are not created equal; each has its pluses and minuses. In the following section, I've outlined the differences among workouts and why some of them may work better for you than others. Rest assured that there is something for everyone here.

When you start any cardiovascular exercise program, it's important to check with your doctor, especially if you have any serious medical conditions, such as high blood pressure, heart problems, lung disease, diabetes, or an orthopedic problem. It's important to make sure you're not compromising your health.

Walking. This is my first choice for most people just starting an exercise program. Everyone can do it, and it can be done almost anywhere. Plus it's easy on the joints and has a low rate of injury. Either outdoor walking or treadmill walking is acceptable, but be sure not to confuse walking for cardiovascular fitness with strolling. You have to get your heart rate *up*. The only downside to walking is that as you get fitter, it becomes harder to get continued improvements in cardiovascular conditioning and weight loss. You may need to add some jogging or mix in another type of aerobic workout to increase the difficulty. If you walk on a treadmill, raising the grade significantly, even all the way up to 15 percent, is another good way to intensify the challenge.

Hiking. Whether you can hike often enough to meet your cardio requirements will depend on where you live, but if you live in an area where hiking is easily accessible, take advantage of it. You burn more calories and use your muscles in different ways when walking up and down hills than you do on flat ground.

Jogging/Running. It's hard to beat jogging (slow running) and running for quick results, and if you can, I recommend that you do it once or twice a week. But it also places a lot of stress on your body. Many runners get sidelined with injuries, especially overuse injuries. If you're going to choose jogging or running, don't do it more than three days per week and make sure you mix it up with something that uses different muscles or is easier on the body (such as cycling).

Stair Climbing. Stair-stepping machines provide a good workout, though they're getting harder to find in gyms these days, perhaps because many people used them exclusively, didn't cross train, and ended up with overuse injuries. When you use a step machine, the stepper supports some of your weight so you're not moving all of your body weight, which is key to getting an optimal cardiovascular workout. For an even better aerobic workout, try running or walking up real stairs. It can get tedious, but if you're up for it and don't have knee problems, it's a great way to get aerobically fit. If your neighborhood doesn't have any staircases, try the bleachers at a local school stadium.

Cycling. Cycling is fun, and as long as you challenge yourself, it will give you a good cardiovascular workout. I recommend that if you choose outdoor cycling as your main cardiovascular exercise, you double the duration of your workout. The bike gives your body a lot of assistance, so you need to double down to get the same results that you might get from, say, running or even brisk walking. My advice, too, is don't depend solely on the bike. The low-impact nature of the sport means that you don't stress the bones enough to prevent bone loss, and some studies have shown that cyclists can be as or even more prone to bone loss than inactive individuals.

Elliptical exercise. I'm a big fan of this type of exercise because it gets your heart rate up with minimal impact and it works both the upper and lower body. While the elliptical trainer gives you a great cardiovascular workout, it doesn't feel punishing, which is why a lot of people who typically don't like machines do well with elliptical exercise. The best elliptical trainers are the ones that allow you to use your arms and require you to lift your legs in a running-type motion. Octane Fitness makes a great one (www.octanefitness.com).

Stationary cycling. Just about every gym has a stationary bike and it can give you a good aerobic workout—as long as you pedal vigorously. Many people tend to take it too easy on stationary bikes. Take a page from spinning classes (see below) and try pedaling to music, which may help you pedal a little faster, and up the resistance to make the workout more challenging. Stationary bikes support your weight, so you typically don't get as good a workout as on other types of machines, and they don't provide the kind of impact that keeps bones strong. If you have a back problem, you might try a recumbent stationary bike; however, you can pedal these without much effort, so be sure you're working at a 7 or 8 on the Perceived Exertion Scale (page 58). For at-home workouts, you can also purchase a trainer apparatus that allows you to turn your regular bike into a stationary one.

Stationary rowing. A great upper and lower body workout as long as you do it at a vigorous pace, rowing is virtually nonimpact. There can be a tedium factor with stationary rowing, but if you're at a gym you can avoid boredom by doing part of your workout on the rower and part on another (or even more than one) machine. For instance, if your workout is forty minutes long, you might do only the first ten minutes on the rower.

Cardio class. Fitness instructors are really getting creative these days so if you like moving to music, I urge you to check out the schedule at your local gym or exercise studio. Zumba, Afro-Brazilian dance, hip-hop, and cardio fusion are just some of the latest choices on the aerobic menu. The advantage of going to a fitness center is that you'll find a variety of classes, but if you take only one of them regularly, it may become less challenging with time. Many instructors don't vary their routines. In addition, if this is your only cardio workout, you're putting yourself at risk for an overuse injury.

Spinning. These classes are typically done to invigorating music so they tend to be very motivating. The music, though, is just part of what makes the classes fun and encourages you to work hard. The instructor makes a huge difference, so make sure you find a good one. The only downside to spinning is that when a bike supports your weight, you don't get quite as good a workout as when you're on the ground, and like regular cycling it doesn't do much to help keep your bones strong. However, you can increase the resistance on spinning bikes, which helps compensate for the difference the bike's support makes, and many spinning instructors have you stand as you pedal, which puts some beneficial stress on your bones (though not as much as, say, jogging).

Swimming. While swimming works all your muscles, it lends itself to moving slowly — most people don't swim fast enough to get the aerobic benefits they need. Also, traditionally, vigorous cardiovascular activity reduces your appetite, probably by heating up your body. Swimming doesn't raise your body temperature to the same degree as other types of cardiovascular exercise (the water helps cool you down), so you may not get the appetite-reducing benefit of exercise. Worse, swimming can actually stimulate your appetite. If you have trouble getting your speed up on your own, consider joining a masters swimming workout, where you'll have a coach to put you through the paces.

DVD-led aerobic workouts and Wii Fit. Pop in the disk and you're off; in most cases you don't even need a lot of room to exercise. The majority of DVD workouts also include a warm-up and cool-down segment, which is a plus. They're also great for travel; many hotels have DVD players in the rooms. My only caveat: be careful that you don't end up with an overuse injury from doing the same thing day after day. A DVD program isn't going to change, so you're going to be working the same muscles in the same way over and over again. For best and safest results, have several DVDs in your arsenal and alternate them. If you choose the Wii, make sure that you select a Wii program that is expressly for cardio.

Jumping rope. This is a very inexpensive and, if you're proficient, excellent way to get fit. You can also take a jump rope with you wherever you go. However, it can be pretty tough on the body and requires the ability to zone out; otherwise it can get pretty boring. You may want to spend just a few minutes jumping rope, then combine it with another activity for a longer cardio workout. Note that it's not a great choice for beginners. If you do decide to jump rope, be cautious about the surface you jump on. Concrete is too hard on the body, and asphalt is only slightly better. The best surface is a wood floor or aerobic flooring (a shock-absorbing surface). You can buy aerobic flooring in small dimensions and use it to jump rope on.

Outdoor rowing/canoeing/kayaking/stand-up paddling. This is another type of exercise that's fantastic if you can do it at a high and continuous level. Stand-up paddling in particular is great for building core and overall strength as you build aerobic endurance. But you can't just go out and paddle around and expect to see cardiovascular improvements. Choose it only if you can turn it into a vigorous, sustainable workout. Also be aware that rowing allows you to use your whole body, whereas canoeing and kayaking are more upper-body workouts.

Ice-skating and in-line skating. Obviously, you need to have a rink nearby to make ice-skating work, and you also have to skate continuously to make the workout effective, which can sometimes be hard to do. Yet if you can manage to hit the right level of exertion and you love going to the rink, ice-skating is a very good form of exercise. In-line skating can be a lot more convenient than ice-skating and has many of the same benefits.

Cross-country skiing. This is one of the few workouts that vigorously challenges both the upper and lower body. What's more, it places little stress on the muscles, joints, and ligaments. Of course, you're beholden to the weather, which can be a drawback. Always have a back-up activity in mind so that you're not left out in the cold if it doesn't snow.

Downhill skiing. To make downhill skiing a sustained cardiovascular activity (twenty minutes minimum) you'll have to find some long runs. But if you can do it, it's excellent for aerobic training and great conditioning for your legs.

Horseback riding. Most people don't think of horseback riding as an aerobic activity, but if you do it vigorously it requires a lot of heart and lung power.

The Perceived Exertion Scale

The optimum level of exertion is a 7 or 8. It may take a while for you to work up to this intensity—or to maintain it for any length of time—but it will come. If you can't hit that pace right off the bat, start at a lower level of exertion and try to exercise at a 7 for a minute or two before moving back to your more comfortable pace. Build on that, adding a minute as you can so that you eventually work up to a whole workout at level 7 or 8.

0 This is the way you feel at rest. There is no fatigue, and your breathing is not elevated.

1 This is how you'd feel while working at your desk or reading. There is no fatigue, and your breathing is normal.

2 This is what you'd feel like when you're getting dressed. There is little or no feeling of fatigue, and your breathing is still normal.

3 This is how you'd feel while walking slowly across the room to turn on the TV. You may feel a little fatigued and you may be aware of your breathing, but it is still slow and natural. You also might feel this way in the beginning of an exercise session.

4 This is the way you would feel if you were walking slowly outside. There is a slight feeling of fatigue and your breathing is slightly elevated but comfortable. You should experience this level during the initial stages of your warm-up.

5 This is how you'd feel while walking somewhere at a normal pace. You're aware of your breathing, which is now deeper, and there is a slight feeling of fatigue. You should experience this level at the end of your warm-up.

6 This is how you'd feel if you were hurrying to an appointment for which you were late. There is a feeling of fatigue, but you know you can maintain this

level of exertion. Your breathing is deep, and you're aware of it. This is how you should feel as you transition from warm-up to your regular exercise session.

7   This is how you'd feel if you were exercising at moderate to moderately high intensity. There's a feeling of fatigue, but you're sure you can maintain this level for the rest of your exercise session. Your breathing is deep, and you're aware of it. You could carry on a conversation but would probably choose not to do so. You should try to maintain this level during your workouts.

8   This is how you should feel when you're exercising vigorously at moderately high intensity. You're feeling fatigued, and if you asked yourself if you could continue for the remainder of your exercise session, your answer would be that you think you could but you're not sure. You're on the edge, but you can maintain the pace, at least for a fairly good while. Your breathing is very deep, and though you could still carry on a conversation, you don't feel like it. You should try to exercise at this level only after you're feeling comfortable enough at level 7. Many people see rapid results at this level.

9   This is what you'd feel like if you were exercising very, very vigorously. You'd definitely feel fatigued, and you probably wouldn't be able to maintain this high-intensity level for very long. Your breathing is very labored, and it would be very difficult to carry on a conversation. If you're doing interval training, you may hit this level for short periods of time, but it's not a level that you can or need to stay at for a lengthy duration.

10 This level is all-out exercise, so difficult that you couldn't maintain it for very long. Hence, there's no benefit to it.

STRENGTH-TRAINING EXERCISES

The majority of these exercises can be done with dumbbells, but when you get to Level III, some are done on the type of weight machines you find in gyms. If you don't have access to weight machines, skip those exercises.

1. Heel Raise

Stretches and strengthens the calves and helps prevent shin splints.

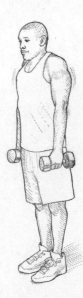

- Stand on a board approximately 2 inches thick by 36 inches long, or any other stable surface raised a few inches off the ground. (If necessary, you can also do this without a board.) Place the ball of each foot on the raised area, with heels on the floor. Keep feet about 12 inches apart; knees are straight, but not locked.

- Inhale and slowly raise heels as high as you can and hold for 1 second before slowly lowering down to starting position, exhaling as you go. Do 15 times for each set.

2. Shrug Roll

Helps stabilize the shoulders (deltoids)/rotator cuffs.

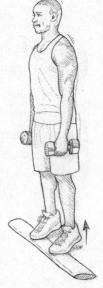

- Stand up straight, feet a little apart and arms at your sides. Inhale, shrug shoulders up toward your ears as high as they can go. Pause for a second in this position, then exhale and roll shoulders back while squeezing your shoulder blades together. Pause for a second in midsqueeze, then drop shoulders back to the starting position. Do 10 times for each set.

3. Squat

Works the upper legs (quadriceps, hamstrings).

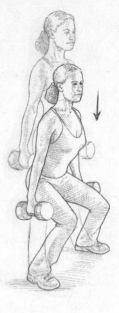

- Stand with feet slightly wider than shoulder-width apart, your back straight, head up, and toes and knees pointed slightly out. There should be a slight bend in your knees. Hold a dumbbell in each hand, your arms at your sides and palms facing inward.

- Contract your abdominal muscles. Bend your knees, gradually lowering your body (as if you were going to sit in a chair) until your thighs are almost parallel with the floor; never let them go lower than parallel with the floor. Pause for a second, then push up from your heels and gradually return to starting position. Control your movements throughout the exercise, inhaling on the way down, exhaling on the way up. Do 8 to 10 repetitions for each set.

4. Chest Press

Works the chest and back of upper arms (pectoralis major, pectoralis minor, triceps).

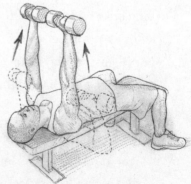

- Lie on your back on a bench with your knees bent and your feet on the floor. Keep your back flat against the bench, with little or no arch. Hold a dumbbell in each hand slightly above chest level, elbows bent out to the side and your palms facing away from you.

- Contract your abdominal muscles. Gradually raise the dumbbells until your arms are fully extended above your chest. Do not hyperextend your elbows. Pause for a second, then gradually return dumbbells to starting position. Control your movements throughout the exercise, exhaling while raising the dumbbells and inhaling on the return. Do 8 to 10 repetitions for each set.

5. Biceps Curl

Works the upper arms (biceps).

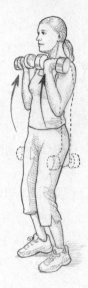

- Stand with your feet slightly apart and knees slightly bent. Hold a dumbbell in each hand, your arms at your sides, palms facing inward.

- Contract your abdominals. Curl the dumbbells up to your shoulder while twisting your palms so that they are facing you at top of move. Pause for a second and then gradually lower dumbbells to starting position. Control movements throughout the exercise, exhaling while lifting the dumbbells up and inhaling on the return. Do 8 to 10 repetitions for each set.

6. Thumbs Down

Works the shoulders (deltoids)/rotator cuffs.

- Stand erect with your feet shoulder-width apart. Holding a dumbbell in each hand in front of your thighs, rotate your arms inward so that your thumbs touch your thighs. Keep your knees slightly bent.

- Contract your abdominal muscles. With your arms straight (but not hyperextended) raise both dumbbells up in front of you to shoulder height while still keeping your thumbs down and arms rotated inward. Pause for a split second, then return to the starting position. Control your movements throughout the entire exercise, exhaling as you raise the dumbbells and inhaling on the way down. Do 8 to 10 repetitions for each set.

7. Lunge

Works the legs (quadriceps, hamstrings, calves).

- Stand with your feet shoulder-width apart, your back straight, head up, and knees slightly bent. Hold a dumbbell in each hand, your arms at your sides and palms facing inward.

- Contract your abdominal muscles. Step forward with your right foot and bend both knees so that your front thigh becomes parallel to the floor. Your front knee should be directly above your ankle, never beyond it. Pause for a second and return to the starting position by pushing off from your front foot. Control your movement throughout the exercise, inhaling as you step forward, exhaling on the return. Do 8 to 10 repetitions, then switch sides. Do another 8 to 10 repetitions for each set.

8. One-Arm Row

Works the back and shoulders (deltoids).

- Kneel on a bench with your right arm supporting your weight. Hold a dumbbell in your left hand with your arm naturally hanging down, palm facing in toward your side.

- Contract your abdominal muscles. Bend your left elbow and gradually raise the dumbbell up to about chest height. Your elbow should be kept high and finish above your shoulder. Pause for a split second, then return to the starting position. Control your movements throughout the entire exercise, exhaling as you raise the dumbbell and inhaling as you return to the starting position. Do 8 to 10 repetitions; switch sides. Do another 8 to 10 repetitions for each set.

9. Dumbbell Fly

Works the chest (pectoralis major, pectoralis minor).

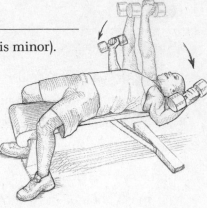

- Lie on your back on a bench with your knees bent and your feet flat on the floor. Keep your back flat against the bench, with little or no arch, and your arms fully extended but not hyperextended above your chest and perpendicular to the floor. Hold a dumbbell in each hand, palms facing inward.

- Contract your abdominal muscles. Gradually lower dumbbells out to the side, keeping elbows slightly bent throughout the exercise. Continue until upper arms are parallel with floor. Pause for a second, then gradually return to starting position. Control movements throughout the exercise, exhaling while lowering the dumbbells and inhaling on the return. Do 8 to 10 repetitions for each set.

10. Triceps Extension

Works the backs of upper arms (triceps).

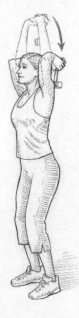

- Stand with your feet slightly apart and your knees slightly bent. Raise one dumbbell above your head and clasp it with both hands, fingers intertwined. Your arms should be fully extended but not hyperextended.

- Contract your abdominal muscles. Gradually bend your elbows and lower the dumbbell back behind your head and neck. Keep your upper arms in place and continue lowering the weight until your forearms are parallel to floor. Pause for a second, then gradually raise the dumbbell to starting position. Control movements throughout the exercise, inhaling while lowering the dumbbell and exhaling while raising it back up. Do 8 to 10 repetitions for each set.

11. Shoulder Press

Works the shoulders (deltoids).

- Sit upright on a chair or slightly slanted if using an incline bench, with your back supported and your feet flat on the floor. Keep your back flat against the back of the chair or bench, with little or no arch. Hold a dumbbell in each hand slightly above shoulder level and with your palms facing away from you, elbows out to the side.

- Contract your abdominals. Keeping palms facing away from you, raise the dumbbells up and inward until the ends of dumbbells are nearly touching each other and are directly overhead. Do not hyperextend your elbows. Pause for a second, then gradually lower the dumbbells to starting position. Control your movements throughout the exercise, exhaling while raising the dumbbells and inhaling on the return. Do 8 to 10 repetitions for each set.

12. External Rotation

Works the shoulders (deltoids)/rotator cuffs.

- Lie on a mat on your left side with your left arm bent and your head resting in your hand. Hold a dumbbell in your right hand, your right arm bent at a 90-degree angle and your elbow resting on your side, slightly above your hip. Rest the weight on the floor.

- Contract your abdominal muscles. Keeping your elbow resting on your side, slowly raise the weight up until it is pointed at the ceiling or as high as your range of motion allows. Pause for a split second at the top before gradually lowering the dumbbell. Control your movements throughout the entire exercise, exhaling as you raise the dumbbell and inhaling on the way down. Do 8 to 10 repetitions; switch sides. Do another 8 to 10 repetitions for each set.

13. Leg Extension (machine only)

Works the front of the legs (quadriceps).

■ Sit on the machine's seat with your body erect and your back firmly against the seat. Adjust the leg arm of the machine so that your knees are centered with the pivot point. The leg pad should be adjusted so that it rests comfortably above your feet. With your thighs parallel to each other and 4 to 5 inches of space between your knees, legs straight but not locked, point your toes straight up or with a slight pitch forward. Grasp the handholds firmly and look straight ahead.

■ Contract your abdominal muscles. Extend your legs completely without locking your knees. Pause for a split second before returning the weight to the starting position. Pause for a split second before starting the next repetition. Control your movements throughout the entire exercise, exhaling as you extend your legs and inhaling as you return to starting position. Do 8 to 10 repetitions for each set.

14. Leg Curl (machine only)

Works the back of the legs (hamstrings).

- Sit on the machine's seat with your body erect and your back firmly against the seat. Adjust the leg arm of the machine so that your knees are centered with the pivot point. The leg pad should be adjusted so that it rests comfortably on the back of the leg, just above the Achilles tendon. Lower the thigh stabilization pad to fit snugly across the thighs. With your thighs parallel to each other and 4 to 5 inches of space between your knees, legs straight but not locked, point your toes straight up or with a slight pitch forward. Grasp the handholds firmly and look straight ahead.

- Contract your abdominal muscles. Bend your knees at a 90-degree angle. Pause for a split second, then allow your legs to slowly come back to starting position. Pause for a split second before starting the next repetition. Control your movements throughout the entire exercise, exhaling as you bend your legs and inhaling as you return to starting position. Do 8 to 10 repetitions for each set.

15. Lateral Raise

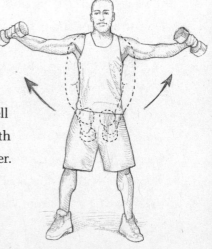

Works the shoulders (deltoids)/rotator cuffs.

- Stand erect with your feet shoulder width apart, your arms down, and a slight bend in your elbows. Hold a dumbbell in each hand, one in front of each thigh with your palms facing inward toward each other. Keep your knees slightly bent.

- Contract your abdominal muscles. Raise each dumbbell out to the side in a semicircular motion until your arms are parallel with the floor. Pause for a split second before gradually lowering the dumbbells to the starting position. Control your movements throughout the entire exercise, exhaling as you raise the dumbbells and inhaling as you return to starting position. Do 8 to 10 repetitions for each set.

16. Upright Row

Works the shoulders (deltoids).

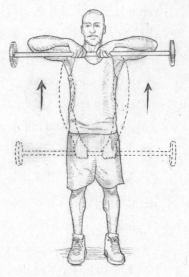

- Stand with your feet shoulder-width apart, your arms straight and your torso erect. Using an overhand grip, hold a barbell (preferred for this exercise) or dumbbells in your hands, allowing them to rest lightly on your thighs (if using a barbell, grip the bar with hands 2 to 4 inches apart).

- Contract your abdominal muscles. With your elbows pointed outward, gradually pull the weights upward along your abdomen and chest until your elbows reach shoulder height. Exhale as the weights reach your shoulders, pause for a split second, and inhale as you gradually lower the weights to starting position. Control your movements as you go. Do 8 to 10 repetitions for each set.

17. Incline Chest Press (requires incline board)

Works the upper chest and back of upper arms (triceps).

- Lie with your back flat against an incline bench with little or no arch in your back. Keep your knees bent and feet flat on the floor. Bend your elbows and hold a dumbbell in each hand slightly above chest level, palms facing away from you.

- Contract your abdominal muscles. Gradually raise both dumbbells up until your arms are fully extended above your chest. Do not hyperextend your elbows. Pause for a split second, then gradually return the dumbbells back to starting position. Control your movements throughout the entire exercise, exhaling as you raise the dumbbells and inhaling on the return. Do 8 to 10 repetitions for each set.

18. Frontal Raise

Works the shoulders (deltoids).

- Stand erect with your feet shoulder-width apart. Hold a dumbbell in each hand with your arms down and your palms facing your thighs. Your closed fingers should be lightly touching your thighs. Keep your knees slightly bent.

- Contract your abdominal muscles. Raise both dumbbells up in front of you to shoulder height. Pause for a split second, then return to starting position. Control your movements throughout the entire exercise, exhaling as you raise the dumbbells and inhaling on the way down. Do 8 to 10 repetitions for each set.

19. Lat Pull-Down (machine only)

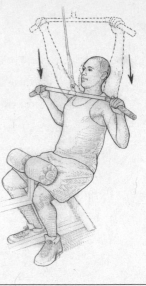

Works the upper back and chest (pectoralis major, pectoralis minor).

▪ While seated (or kneeling if the station has no seat) at a lat pull station, grip the bar using an overhand grip with your hands a few inches wider than shoulder-width apart. Your torso should be slightly tilted backward and your arms extended.

To Keep It Interesting, Exercise Alternatives

There are many different ways to work the same muscles. Every six to eight months, consider changing up the exercises you do. That will keep your workout fresh and challenge your muscles in the same but also slightly different ways. Here are alternatives to the strength-training moves listed on pages 60 to 63. See my website 20YearsYounger.com for more on these exercises.

Instead of Heel Raise:
Heel Raise with Band
Heel to Toe Rock

Instead of Shrug Roll:
Behind-the-Back Barbell Shrug
Calf Raise Shoulder Shrug (machine)
Shrug with Band

Instead of Squat:
Leg Press (machine)
Swiss Ball No-Weight Squat
Wall Sit
One-Legged Step Down

Instead of Chest Press:
Push-Up
Chest Press with Resistance Band
Seated Chest Press (machine)

Instead of Biceps Curl:
Biceps Curl with Bands
Incline Biceps Curl
Hammer Curl
Pull-Ups

Instead of Thumbs Down:
Cross Body with Band

Instead of Lunge:
Multi-Plane Lunge
Walking Lunge

Instead of One-Arm Row:
Back Extensions
Incline Bench Pull
One-Arm Row with Exercise Band

- Contract your abdominal muscles. Pull the bar straight down in front of your face. Pull smoothly, keeping your elbows out and away from your body. Pull the bar past your chin until it lightly touches your upper chest. Pause for a split second, then return to the starting position. Control your movements throughout the entire exercise, exhaling as the bar approaches your chest and inhaling as you release back to starting position. Do 8 to 10 repetitions for each set.

Instead of Dumbbell Fly

Fly (machine)

Disk Fly

Fly with Exercise Band

Instead of Triceps Extension:

Dip

Cable Push Down (machine)

Plank Up

Instead of External Rotation:

Dumbbell Rotation with Arm
  Abduction

External Rotation with Band

External Rotation Double-Handed

Instead of Leg Extension:

Single-Leg Quad Raise

Chair Straight-Leg Extension

Instead of Leg Curl:

Hamstring Roll-In

Butt Blaster

Bridge

Instead of Lateral Raise:

Incline Lat Raise on Ball

Bent-Arm Lateral Raise

Lateral Raise (machine)

Instead of Upright Row:

Double-Arm High Pull

Prone Incline Shoulder Press

Upright Row with Band or Tube

Instead of Incline Chest Press:

Incline Chest Press on Ball

Incline Chest Press with Band

Push-Up on Ball

Instead of Frontal Raise:

Incline Front Raise

Front Raise with Band

Instead of Lat Pull-Down:

Lat Pull-Down with Band

Cable Straight-Arm Pull-Down
  (machine)

Pull-Up

STRETCHES

1. Hamstring Stretch

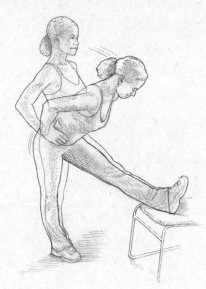

- Stand with one foot propped up on a step or on a chair in front of you, legs straight. Place hands on hips, making sure you're stable. Keep the leg that is lifted straight and slowly bend your torso toward your toes, keeping your back straight until you feel a stretch in the back of your legs (hamstrings). Breathe evenly as you stay in the stretch. Hold for 5 seconds (no bouncing) and relax for another 5 seconds. Repeat on each leg 3 to 5 times.

2. Quadriceps Stretch

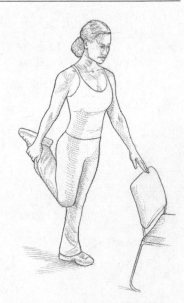

- Standing, hold on to the back of a chair with your left hand. Bend your right knee behind you and grab your right ankle with your right hand. Bring your heel toward your buttocks until you feel a little tension in your thigh. Keep the knee of the other leg slightly bent. Both knees should be parallel. Breathe evenly as you stay in the stretch. Hold for 5 seconds, relax for 5 seconds, and continue this way for 3 or 4 stretches. Repeat on the other side.

3. Upper Calf Stretch

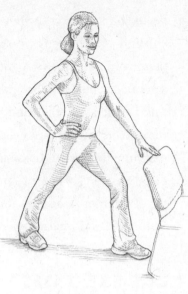

- Standing, hold on to the back of a chair with your left hand while placing the other hand on your right hip. Bend your left leg about 45 degrees and bring your right leg straight out behind you about 3 feet and place your heel on the floor. Your bent left knee should be right above your left foot (not in front of it). If you don't feel the stretch in your right leg, bring the left foot forward a little more. Do not arch your back. Breathe evenly as you stay in the stretch. Hold for 5 seconds, relax for 5 seconds, repeat 2 more times. Then switch legs and repeat.

4. Lower Calf Stretch

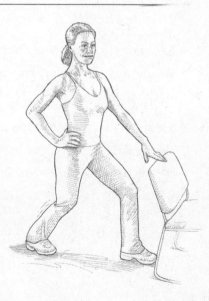

- Standing, hold on to the back of a chair with your left hand. Place your right hand on your hip and slide your right leg straight out behind you about 2 feet, keeping the heel on the ground. Bend both knees and slowly lower your hips toward the floor, keeping both heels on the ground. You should feel gentle tension in the lower calf of your back leg. Breathe evenly as you stay in the stretch. Hold for 5 seconds; relax for 5 seconds; repeat 2 more times. Switch sides.

5. Middle and Lower Back Stretch

- Seated on a chair with your knees apart, hold your arms out in front of you and stretch them forward. Keeping them in this position, gradually bend your torso forward and allow your back to round until you feel a gentle tension in your upper and/or middle back. (At this point, your arms may be between your knees, hands touching the floor if possible.) Breathe evenly as you stay in the stretch. Hold the stretch for 5 seconds, relax for 5 seconds, and repeat 2 more times.

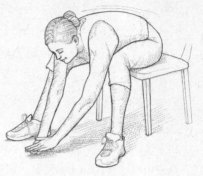

CORE EXERCISES

1. Basic Crunch

- Lie on your back, with knees bent, feet flat on the floor, and heels 12 to 15 inches from your buttocks. Place both your hands behind your neck.

- Let your abs do the work of raising your torso straight up to a 30-to-45-degree angle, but don't curl your body or your back up. Point your chin to the ceiling.

- Hold for 1 second, then lower down. Exhale as you rise up; inhale as you lower down. Do 15 times for each set.

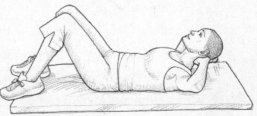

2. Upper Abdominal Crunch

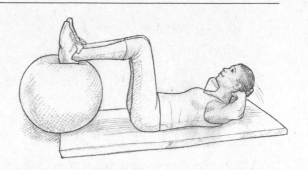

- Lie on your back with your elbows out, hands behind your neck.

- Bend your knees at a 90-degree angle and rest your feet on an exercise ball or chair.

- Raise your torso to a 35-to-45-degree angle and hold for a second.

- Return to starting position. Exhale as you rise up; inhale as you lower down. Do 15 times for each set.

3. Twisting Trunk Curl Crunch

- Lie on your back, with knees bent and heels 12 to 15 inches from your buttocks. Place both hands behind your neck.

- Place your left ankle over your right knee so that your legs form a triangle.

- Let your abs do the work of raising your right shoulder toward your left knee, 8 to 12 inches off the ground. Return to starting position. Exhale as you rise up; inhale as you lower down.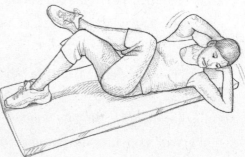

- Do 15 on this side, then switch legs and repeat for another 15 for each set.

4. Alternating Arm and Leg Raise

- Lie on your stomach, facedown, arms stretched out in front of you, with your head supported by a folded towel. (The towel goes under your armpits and under your chin.)

- Raise your right arm and your left leg simultaneously by contracting your abdominal and lower back muscles. Keep your shoulders and pelvis pressed against the floor and your arm and leg straight. Your left arm and right leg should be on the floor.

- Lift to the point at which you feel a gentle tension in the lower back muscles. Pause for a second before going back to starting position. Exhale as you rise up; inhale as you lower down.

- Do 15 times, then repeat on the other side 15 times for each set.

5. Extended Arm Crunch

- Lie face-up on the floor with your knees bent, feet flat on the floor, and your heels 12 to 15 inches from your buttocks. Place one hand behind your neck for support. Extend the other arm straight out so that it is between your knees.

- Contract your abdominal muscles and use them to raise your torso off the floor to a 30-to-45-degree angle. Your chin should go straight up toward the ceiling with no rolling of your neck. Pause for a split second before returning to starting position. Exhale as you rise up; inhale as you lower down.

- Do 15 for each set.

6. Vertical Leg Crunch

- Lie face-up on the floor with your legs straight up, perpendicular to the ground, knees bent slightly. Place your palms lightly behind your neck.

- Contract your abdominal muscles and use them to raise your torso off the floor to a 30-to-45-degree angle. Your chin should go straight up toward the ceiling with no rolling of your neck. Pause for a split second before returning to starting position. Exhale as you rise up; inhale as you lower down.

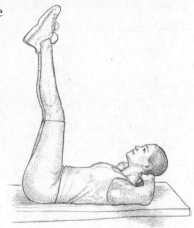

- Do 15 for each set.

7. The Reverse Trunk Curl

- Lie on your back, with your legs straight up, perpendicular to the ground, knees bent slightly. Place your palms facedown and at your sides.

- Keep your back — including your shoulder blades — as flat as possible on the floor. Contract your abdominal muscles and curl up your pelvis. This will raise your legs up higher toward the ceiling. Hips should be 3 to 5 inches off the floor. Pelvis and buttocks should be fairly relaxed; it's your abdominal muscles doing the work. Exhale as you contract your abs and hold for 1 second. Inhale on the way down. Do 15 for each set.

8. Incline Sit-Up (requires incline board)

- Lie face-up on an incline board with your knees bent, feet hooked under the board's leg pads. Place your hands behind your neck with your elbows out to the side. Your back should be flat against the pad of the board and your feet locked under the footholds.

- Contract your abdominal muscles and use them to raise your torso to a 35-to-45-degree angle. Your chin should point straight up toward the ceiling; don't let your neck roll as you rise up, and keep your shoulders square. Pause for a second before returning to starting position. Exhale as you rise up; inhale as you lower down.

- Do 15 for each set.

- Increasing the height of the incline board will increase the challenge. Try doing each set on a different setting.

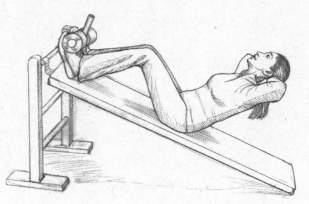

LIFETIME SPORTS AND RECREATIONAL ACTIVITIES

Some of these sports and activities are especially good for balance, some are especially good for hand-eye coordination, and some are good for both. A few of them are simply excellent ways to get more physical and social activity into your life.

Archery*

Badminton*†

Baseball/softball*

Basketball*†

Bike riding†

Bocce*†

BOSU Ball/balance boards†

Bowling*†

Boxing/punching speed bag*

Canoeing

Climbing (rock/wall)*†

Cricket*

Croquet*

Dancing†

Darts*

Fishing

Football*

Frisbee*

Gardening/yardwork

Golf*†

Gymnastics†

Hockey (roller or ice)*†

Hopscotch†

Horseback riding†

Horseshoes*

Hunting*

Ice-skating†

In-line skating†

Jacks*

Jump rope†

Karate/martial arts†

Kayaking

Kiteboarding†

Lacrosse/field hockey*

Lawn bowling*

Mountain biking†

Netball*

Paddleboarding†

Pilates†

Ping-Pong*

Playing catch (with football, baseball)*

Plyometrics†

Polo*

Quoits*

Racquet sports (squash, racquetball, handball)*†

River rafting†

Rugby*

Sailing†

Shuffleboard*

Skiing/snowboarding†

Step aerobics†

Surfing†

Swimming

Tai chi†

Tennis*†

Volleyball*†

Wake boarding†

Walking†

Water aerobics

Water polo*

Water skiing†

Wind surfing†

Wrestling†

Yoga†

Especially good for hand-eye coordination

†*Especially good for balance*

CHAPTER 3

Lifelong, Life-Lengthening Eating

WHEN I WAS ON THE CROSS-COUNTRY BIKE RIDE I described earlier in the book and pulled into Chicago, I got to ride right onto the set of *The Oprah Winfrey Show* while it was in the middle of taping. I didn't even get off the bike (a surprise guest, just passing through!) but stopped to chat with Oprah. "Wow," she said, "I hear you're drinking gallons of orange juice. Is it true you're eating eight to nine thousand calories a day? That's my dream." "I know it is," I replied, and I couldn't resist adding, "but your dream doesn't involve riding a hundred miles a day. That's you're biggest nightmare!"

Who wouldn't like to eat all that they wanted every day? Maybe not eight to nine thousand calories, but it would be nice to eat whatever you felt like without any worries about the repercussions. Because of my profession people often expect me to be a perfect eater. I'll go out with friends or business associates and besides watching every morsel I put in *my* mouth, they'll become very self-conscious about what they're ordering. But not only do I enjoy food, I like to see other people enjoying food, too.

Once when I was appearing on a local morning show, I talked with a variety of other interesting guests in the greenroom of the television station as we waited for our respective turns in front of the camera. When I heard my name called, I headed out onto the stage.

Earlier, I had noticed that there was a huge tray of doughnuts sitting on a table in the middle of the greenroom. While I was chatting with everyone, nobody had touched them, but when I came back into the room after my appearance, I noticed there wasn't so much as a crumb left. It looked like someone had taken a vacuum cleaner to the tray. My publicist, who had accompanied me to the TV station and saw me looking at the tray, began to laugh. "The second you walked out, they dove into those doughnuts like there was no tomorrow." Obviously, they had been too intimidated to eat in front of me.

The truth is, I love to eat a variety of foods and I love dessert (okay, maybe I don't eat doughnuts, but I find it difficult to turn down any type of pie). I'm human. I battle cravings just like anyone else. Over the years, I've certainly improved my diet. I eat better now than I did in my twenties and thirties, but that's because I have to. You just can't get away with as much when you get older, and if you do make the effort to eat more moderately and nutritiously, there are plenty of life-lengthening and anti-aging benefits to be had.

It's estimated that up to a third of cancer cases, half of heart disease cases, and up to 90 percent of cases of type 2 diabetes are entirely related to less-than-healthy diets as well as how much body fat a person is carrying around. On the flip side, many societies known for their longevity boast diets that are nutrient-rich and far more reasonable in calories than those diets associated with disease. The evidence that you have a greater likelihood of living a longer, higher-quality life if you eat well and moderately is undeniable.

One thing we know about the aging process is that it is accompanied by a slowdown in the metabolic rate (the rate at which you burn calories). As I explained in the previous chapter, exercise can go a long way toward preventing that slowdown; however, most people have to be more careful about how many calories they take in once they approach their forties, or they gain unwanted pounds. I wish I could say that eating however much you want is one of the privileges of aging, but in fact you need to stay extra vigilant about calories as you grow older. There's even some intriguing research, which I'll discuss on page 119, showing that cutting way back on calories can extend your life.

At least as important as the quantity of your food is the quality of your food. There are, of course, the basic building blocks of a nutritious diet: healthy fats, high-quality protein, whole grains, fruits and vegetables. But beyond that, there are also certain foods known to have potent antioxidant powers capable of helping to reduce inflammation and disarm cancer-causing agents, as well as foods that can help lower cholesterol, preserve bone, and keep your brain sharp. Integrate these into your diet and you can greatly enhance your ability to counter various aspects of the aging process.

On the following pages, you'll find an anti-aging eating plan based on all the tenets I just mentioned: don't eat too much, build your diet on healthy staples, and accent it with superfoods. In addition, Tufts researcher Diane L. McKay will weigh in on supplements and how to fill in any potential gaps in your nutrient needs.

EATING FOR HEALTH AND LONGEVITY

Thanks to a whole body of research looking at the connection between certain types of diets and longevity as well as how particular foods affect disease risk factors, we know how to define anti-aging eating. For instance, several epidemiological studies have found that the traditional diets of people living in Mediterranean countries and islands off Japan (Okinawa) seem to confer amazing life-lengthening benefits. Other studies have found that when groups of certain foods are included in a healthy diet, they work together to lower the risk of heart disease. We also now have a lot of information about superfoods, foods from every category that have high levels of disease-fighting compounds and/or have been shown to exact some beneficial changes in the body.

The 20 Years Younger Diet draws from all these sources, but before I tell you more about it, a little background on three of the diets that in part inspired this plan is in order.

The Okinawan Diet is based on research looking at the eating habits and life span of the inhabitants of the Ryukyu Islands (Okinawa is only one of the 161 islands in this string off the coast of Japan, but because it's the largest, its name is used comprehensively). It's well known that Japanese people have half the heart disease rate and about a quarter of the breast and prostate cancer rate as Americans. They also have lower rates of diabetes and Alzheimer's-related dementia. But in Okinawa, the rates for all these chronic diseases are even *lower.* Okinawa also has the largest concentration of centenarians — people age one hundred or older — of anywhere in the world.

Their secret? When Okinawans leave Japan and immigrate to the United States or other countries with a Western-style diet, they gradually, with each succeeding generation, take on a similar risk for chronic disease as everyone else living in that country. "So these people aren't living longer because they have such fabulous genes," says D. Craig Willcox, MHSc, PhD, a professor at Okinawa International University and author of *The Okinawa Program.* "They're living longer because they eat a healthy diet, and stay active and lean." As co-principal investigator of the Okinawa Centenarian Study, Willcox, along with his twin brother, Bradley Willcox, MD, a clinical associate professor at the University of Hawaii, has been tracking the habits of the age-defying Okinawans.

The elderly Okinawans studied by the Willcoxes ate a diet fairly high in carbohydrates, but their carbohydrates came mostly from vegetables and whole grains plus a little fruit (in other words, they weren't packing away lots of baked goods and other junky carbs). They also ate a lot of tofu — even more than in other parts of Japan — and their other protein mainstay was fish. Red meat wasn't regularly on the menu, and when it was, it was generally used as a garnish rather than as the main dish. The types of fat the elderly Okinawans consumed were healthful, something else that set them apart from typical American eaters. Dr. Willcox sums it up. "The reason this way of eating works is because it douses your body with protective phytoactive plant compounds while minimizing the unhealthy stuff like saturated fat, trans fat, white flour and heavily processed foods. In the United States, we eat exactly the opposite way." Another major difference: Okinawans eat about 1,900 calories per day compared to about 2,500 for the average American. What's more, those within the Okinawan population who eat about 15 percent less than average have the longest lives.

The life span of people in Greece and many of the other countries along the Mediterranean Sea rivals that of the Okinawans. The diets in the different countries ringing the Mediterranean aren't identical—for instance, pasta is a staple in Italy, whereas rice and potatoes are more popular in Greece—but they have a lot in common. You might hear their way of eating referred to as the "Mediterranean diet," but given the differences I think it's more appropriate to call it the Mediterranean style of eating. And when I talk about this style of eating, I'm talking about the traditional pattern, no matter which country, of eating plenty of olive oil, a variety of whole grains, lots of fruits and vegetables, and moderate amounts of high-protein foods, mainly fish, with little meat.

There are many differences between the Mediterranean-Style Diet and the Okinawan Diet. They incorporate different types of oils and different fruits and vegetables, and the Okinawans eat no dairy products. But both diets offer similar benefits. Mediterranean countries such as Spain, Italy, and France have about half the rate of death due to heart disease as the United States. And if you already have heart disease, switching over to a Mediterranean-style diet is proving to be a potentially lifesaving move. The Lyon Heart Study of French men and women who'd had one heart attack found that those who followed a Mediterranean-style diet for four years had a 50 to 70 percent lower risk of having a second heart attack than those who followed a diet that was closer to an American diet.

One reason the Mediterranean-Style Diet lowers the risk of heart disease is that it reduces cholesterol, inflammation, and the likelihood of getting type 2 diabetes (diabetes doubles or triples heart disease risk). People who switch to the Mediterranean way of eating lose more weight and have better blood sugar control, two risk factors for diabetes. Followers of the Mediterranean-Style Diet also have lower rates of colorectal, breast, prostate, pancreatic, and endometrial cancers, and a few studies suggest that the diet may even help prevent age-related brain deterioration.

One study tracking older New York for four years found that those who closely adhered to a Mediterranean pattern of eating were 40 percent less likely to develop Alzheimer's disease. French researchers have also found that

How the Anti-Aging Diets Stack Up

The Okinawan and Mediterranean-Style Diets have many similarities—but some notable differences, too. The most significant difference is the quantity of fat in the diets; the Mediterranean-Style Diet allows for quite a bit more. Yet perhaps because the fat eaten in most Mediterranean countries tends to be heart-healthy olive oil, the excess fat doesn't seem to create a problem. Read on to compare and contrast the other differences.

	Mediterranean-Style Diet	Okinawan Diet
percent of calories from carbohydrates	45 to 50	58
percent of calories from protein	15	15
percent of calories from fat	30 to 40	27
percent of calories from saturated fat	7	7
fruits	berries, melons, citrus, apples, pears, grapes, apricots	papaya, pineapple, mangoes, guava, bananas, watermelon, passion fruit, shikwasa (lemon)
vegetables	tomatoes, salad greens, sweet peppers, fennel, eggplant, onions, garlic, purslane	bitter melon, seaweed, shiitake mushrooms, burdock, eggplant, okra, broccoli, carrots, pumpkin, green papaya
herbs	basil, rosemary, thyme, oregano	fennel seeds, turmeric, hot peppers, mugwort, basil, aloe
grains and starchy vegetables	bulgur wheat, whole grain bread, polenta, brown rice, pasta, chickpeas, cannellini beans, lentils	sweet potato, brown rice, buckwheat noodles
high-protein foods	chicken, duck, pigeon, quail, rabbit, lamb, anchovy, sardine, mackerel, sea bream, red tuna, eggs	soy, miso, fish (mahi-mahi, banana fish, reef fish, tuna, bonito), lean pork
dairy	yogurt, cheese	not traditionally eaten
fats	olive oil, almonds, hazelnuts, walnuts	canola oil, soy oil
beverages	water, wine (moderate with meals), tea, coffee	water, jasmine tea, beer, awamori (Okinawan sake)

the diet helps overall cognitive performance and memory. "These findings, though preliminary, show that eating a Mediterranean-style diet may not only affect the risk for Alzheimer's disease, but also put the brakes on other forms of cognitive decline," says Catherine Féart, PhD, of Université Victor Segalen in Bordeaux, France, who led the French study. "Because dementia can take decades to develop, and the Mediterranean diet may have a long-term beneficial effect, it seems that this dietary pattern, and its associated lifestyle, is an optimal dietary strategy if you want to protect your health, including your brain."

A third diet with important benefits for anyone attempting to fight aging is called the Portfolio Diet. University of Toronto researchers asked people to include a "portfolio" of cholesterol-lowering foods such as almonds and egg-plant in their diet. Each of the foods had only mild cholesterol-lowering effects on its own, but together they proved to pack a big punch, lowering LDL (bad) cholesterol in the study subjects by 20 percent or more, signifi-cantly cutting the risk of heart disease. These foods — I'll tell you what they are as you go along — are worth working into your diet, too.

Whereas the Portfolio Diet is virtually a vegan diet (it contains a little nonfat milk and yogurt and its creators encourage the use of plant proteins as much as possible), the Mediterranean and Okinawan diets are not vegan or even vegetarian. They're good examples, though, of how judicious con-sumption of animal foods can still be healthy if you also keep other sources of saturated fat to a minimum, moderate your intake of sodium and sugar, and consume lots of fruits and vegetables.

The Portfolio Diet, the Okinawan Diet, and the Mediterranean-Style Diet collectively tell us a lot about anti-aging nutrition. Yet they have drawbacks, too. Chief among them is that, with our American palates, which are used to the melting pot style of eating (a little Chinese one night, a little Italian the next, some Mexican-influenced cuisine the night after that), following any one of those diets to the letter could get tedious. One of the wonderful things about American markets these days (and that includes farmers' markets and the wide range of ethnic markets as well) is that we have an abundance of foods to choose from, many of which fall into the superfoods category that I talked about earlier. I'm all for taking advantage of that abundance as much as possible, and the 20 Years Younger Diet helps you do so while still giving you the benefits of the Portfolio, Okinawan, and Mediterranean-Style way of eating. Beginning on page 225, you'll find two weeks' worth of menus that draw on all three of these anti-aging diets, mixing in a healthy dose of longevity-promoting superfoods and topping it all off with a dash of convenience (no ingredient is too hard to find or difficult to make). It's the perfect marriage of science and pleasurable eating: a nutritious modern meal plan with enough variety to keep it interesting.

The menu plans will give you initial direction, but it's important to be able to create your own healthy menus. The 20 Years Younger Diet guidelines in the following section will help you with that. If you've been eating poorly, you're going to feel the effects of shifting to this cleaner and more nourishing diet immediately. You'll have more energy, your head will feel clearer, and even your skin will look brighter. If you're already eating fairly nutritiously, the recommendations here will help you fine-tune your diet, showing you how to pack it full of the foods we know can help you live longer and age well. I'll also be continually updating the diet on my website, www.20YearsYounger.com.

THE 20 YEARS YOUNGER DIET

One of the keys to successfully changing your eating habits in order to work toward any goal (be it weight loss, a lower cholesterol level, or overall health and longevity) is making rules for yourself. When you have these rules in place, decision-making about food is simply easier. You know what you can and can't eat and how much food you should have on your plate. I'm not saying that you can never deviate from your nutrition rules, but you'll find it considerably easier to stay on track day to day if you have a framework for eating. To that end, here are the guidelines for anti-aging eating. It's a compilation of what to eat and what not to eat, how to work variety into your diet, and how to sprinkle it all liberally with anti-aging superfoods.

The Guidelines

- At each meal, make sure half of your plate is covered with vegetables and/or fruit.

- For as many meals as possible, the starch on your plate should be either a whole grain (such as whole wheat bread or brown rice), potatoes, sweet potatoes, or legumes (like black beans, pinto beans, or lentils). When you opt for potatoes, make sure they're not fried.

- Your high-protein choices should be mostly fish, chicken, or soy (see page 102 for exceptions to the soy recommendation). Eat red meat no more than three times a month.

- Use mostly olive oil and canola oil.

- Avoid partially hydrogenated oils (trans fats — see pages 106 and 114) and limit saturated fat.

- Choose nonfat or 1% milk or yogurt, or calcium- and vitamin D–enriched soy milk.

- Stick to the treat limit for your calorie level (see chart on page 91); that's 150 calories per day of foods high in sugar (like candy) or salty snacks (like chips) if you're taking in 1,700 calories per day; 200 treat calories on the 2,000-calorie diet, and 250 on 2,500 calories. Bear in mind that the meal plans are full of examples of healthier treats.

- Eliminate or severely limit (no more than twice a month) fried food, soda, or other sugary drinks (like heavily sweetened iced tea and juice "drinks" and punches, which contain very little juice). It's okay to have four ounces of 100 percent fruit juice daily as one of your fruit servings, but any more than that counts as part of your treat calorie allowance. If you decide to have a soda or other sugary drink, that counts as treat calories, too.

The Plan

When you look at the plan below, you'll see that it's divided up into food groups. Under each group, you'll find specific serving recommendations — you don't have to follow these to the letter, but as long as you're close, your diet will be longevity-enhancing. I've also included a list of superfoods that represent the best of the best in the group. Superfoods aren't the only foods you can eat in each category, but opt for them as often as possible. Most of the foods on the list are available in your local supermarket or health food store.

The plan is written to include daily calorie levels ranging from 1,500 to 2,500. How many calories are right for you? The "What's My Calorie Level?" chart below will help you figure out where to start, and I'll include a range of servings recommendations under each category of food so you can see how your calorie level plays out in practical terms. Bear in mind that it may take some trial and error for you to find the calorie level that works for you, whether you're trying to shed pounds or just maintain your weight.

If you're going to have to make a lot of changes in your present diet to switch over to this one, you could get overwhelmed. My suggestion: Start by increasing the amount of fruits and vegetables you eat — that alone can have an amazing impact on your health. Do this for a few weeks, then make your next move. Change the fats that you're eating, then after a few weeks try to weed salty snacks and excessive sweets out of your diet. Keep up the steps until you've mastered all the principles of anti-aging eating.

What's My Calorie Level?

Based on your weight, height, age, exercise level, and how fast you tend to burn calories, your daily calorie needs are very individual. Someone of your exact height, weight, age, and gender who exercises just as much as you do might need a few hundred calories more or less per day than you do. So, keeping in mind that the guidelines below are flexible, use them as a starting point. If you're feeling too hungry or are losing weight too fast (or unnecessarily), move up a calorie level. If you're feeling too full or not losing the weight that you need to lose, drop down a calorie level.

If you're...	And your activity level is...	Try this daily calorie level...
A woman maintaining healthy weight	Sedentary	1,500
A woman who wants to lose weight	Sedentary	1,500 or lower
A woman maintaining healthy weight	Level I	1,700
A woman who wants to lose weight	Level I	1,500
A woman maintaining healthy weight	Level II	2,000
A woman who wants to lose weight	Level II	1,700
A woman maintaining healthy weight	Level III	2,500 (possibly higher; see page 221 for ways to add calories)
A woman who wants to lose weight	Level III	2,000
A man maintaining healthy weight	Sedentary	1,700
A man who wants to lose weight	Sedentary	1,700 or lower
A man maintaining healthy weight	Level I	2,000
A man who wants to lose weight	Level I	1,700
A man maintaining healthy weight	Level II	2,500
A man who wants to lose weight	Level II	2,000
A man maintaining healthy weight	Level III	2,500 + (see page 221 for ways to add calories)
A man who wants to lose weight	Level III	2,500

How Much Do I Eat?

Daily Servings According to Your Calorie Intake

Calorie Intake	1,500	1,700	2,000	2,500
Fruit	2	2	3	4
Vegetables	5	6	7	8
Grains/Starchy Vegetables	5	5	6	7
Milk/Yogurt/Soy Milk	2	2	2	3
Protein-Rich Foods	6	6	7	8
Nuts/Seeds	1	1	1	2
Healthy Fats	5	5	6	7
Treat Calories	none	150	200	250

THE 20 YEARS YOUNGER DIET GROCERY LIST

Fruit

2 to 4 servings daily

Serving = a medium-size fruit (like an orange) or half a cup of berries, grapes, or chopped fruit.

Superfruits

ACAI BERRIES, BLUEBERRIES, BLACKBERRIES, STRAWBERRIES, AND RASPBERRIES. Just a handful or two of berries on your cereal or oatmeal in the morning turns breakfast into brain food. Rich in polyphenols, phytonutrients that have anti-inflammatory and antioxidant powers, berry extract has been shown, through animal studies at the USDA Center on Aging Research at Tufts University, to improve memory by protecting brain cells from age-related decline. "We have little housekeepers in the brain called microglia, which clean up the debris that would otherwise interfere with brain cell function," explains Shibu Poulose, PhD, a molecular biologist at the USDA/Tufts lab. "As we age, these housekeepers get sloppy, leaving debris around and even misdirecting their clean-up efforts on healthy cells, damaging them. Our studies indicate that extracts of blueberries, strawberries, and acai berries may restore microglia back to a functioning level." Among berries' other benefits is helping to lower cholesterol. Strawberries and raspberries also contain ellagic acid, a phytochemical that has anticancer properties.

CITRUS. We've long known that lemons, limes, oranges, and grapefruit are rich in vitamin C, good enough reason not only to eat citrus for snacks and desserts but to use it in cooking as well. (Lemon-based salad dressings, fish topped with an orange and onion salsa, and avocado and grapefruit salads are just a few of the ways to work citrus into meals.) Citrus fruits also contain a group of compounds called flavonoids, which are proving to be potent cancer and heart disease fighters. One of these flavonoids, naringenin, found in very high amounts in grapefruit, can stimulate production of SIRT1, an enzyme that appears to slow aging.

POMEGRANATES. Suddenly, pomegranate is everywhere. Pomegranate juices line store shelves, pomegranate extract is infused in tea, dried pomegranates are mixed into cereals and trail mix — you get the picture. Though pomegranate has long been used in traditional medicine in India, Greece, and the Middle East, scientists are now discovering that it holds promise in preventing clogged arteries and protecting against prostate and other types of cancer.

GRAPES. You hear a lot about the health benefits of wine, but what is wine made of? Grapes, and for my money, going right to the source is the best idea. Red and purple grapes get their pigment from anthocyanins, the same beneficial compounds found in blueberries and blackberries. Green grapes are higher in a compound called flavan-3-ols, which fight cancer and protect the nerves. Grapes of all colors may protect against heart disease and are also rich in a number of phytonutrients. The two considered most effective are proanthocyanidins and resveratrol, which has been making a lot of news lately because it's believed to turn on the cells' own survival mechanisms. Some scientists believe it shows promise for the prevention of many age-related conditions, including Parkinson's and Alzheimer's disease, inflammation, diabetes, and cardiovascular disease. Resveratrol is mainly found in the grape skin; proanthocyanidins are found only in the seeds.

Vegetables

4 to 8 servings daily

Serving = 1 cup raw greens such as spinach or lettuce or ½ cup chopped raw or cooked vegetables

RULE OF THUMB: Vary the type and color of your vegetables in order to consume the most phytonutrients, vitamins, and minerals. Have cruciferous vegetables at least three times a week and the others on this list as often as possible.

Supervegetables

CRUCIFEROUS VEGETABLES. Broccoli, brussels sprouts, cabbage, cauliflower, kale, collard greens, mustard greens, and turnip greens are known as cruciferous vegetables. Cruciferous vegetables turn off a lot of people, but maybe that's because they haven't had them prepared properly. In Mediterranean countries, they're often simply sautéed with olive oil instead of steamed, the way they're commonly served here. Sautéing gives them much greater flavor, which is important, because you want to eat as many servings of cruciferous vegetables as you can: They all share cancer-fighting compounds called iso-thiocyanates, which may disable some of the cancer-causing substances in tobacco smoke and help remove carcinogenic substances before they can damage DNA. Sulforaphane, an isothiocyanate found in broccoli, has been shown to stop cancer cells from growing and even kill them.

EGGPLANT (PURPLE SKIN VARIETY). Eggplant is high in viscous fiber — the type that helps trap fat and cholesterol and whisk it out of the body. That's why it's a staple of the cholesterol-lowering Portfolio Diet. Eggplant's purple skin is also a great source of anthocyanins, which give blueberries some of their healing properties. Be careful how you cook eggplant. It sops up oil like a sponge, so pan-frying isn't the healthiest way to prepare it. Instead, slice the eggplant, spray it with oil, and bake it in the oven. You can also bake the entire eggplant in its skin, then peel it afterward.

PURSLANE. You can find this green in farmers' markets in the summer, and it might even be in your backyard, growing alongside your grass. Eaten in some of the Mediterranean countries and in the Middle East as a salad green, it has unusually high amounts of omega-3 fatty acids for a vegetable (see page 107 for more on omega-3s). A 3½-ounce serving (about 2⅓ cup) contains 300 to 400 mg of omega-3, covering about a third of your daily requirement. It's also high in melatonin, which may help you sleep more soundly.

SEAWEED. There are many types of seaweed, and their nutritional attributes vary. Those that show up regularly in Okinawan cuisine include the following:

- *Kombu:* Okinawans use this mild-tasting seaweed to make broth (dashi). It's rich in heart- and bone-protecting magnesium. Like wakame (below), kombu contains fucoidan, an antioxidant that in test-tube studies kills cancer cells.

- *Hijiki (or hiziki):* Rich in both potassium and magnesium, its tender, dark, curly leaves are often part of a seaweed salad mix or served alone as a salad in Japanese restaurants. You can also buy it dried and turn it into a salad at home.

- *Wakame:* Wakame is the green vegetable traditionally swirling around in miso soup. It's rich in manganese (which is part of the body's own antioxidant defense system) and folate (good for the heart and a cancer fighter). The only downside is that it's very high in sodium, which is why the tofu and miso soup on page 267 substitutes kombu or hijiki for wakame.

To find seaweed, check the Asian section of your supermarket or visit an Asian market. You can also buy it online. Bear in mind that seaweed isn't just for cooking. Many markets now carry snack packs of seaweed that you can eat just like crackers (though with far fewer calories).

MUSHROOMS. We've known for a while that mushrooms have a lot going for them — B vitamins, copper, and phytonutrients that boost immunity and help prevent plaque formation in arteries — but grocery stores are now also starting to carry mushrooms that are rich in vitamin D. Since vitamin D is hard to get from food, this is big news. The mushrooms are exposed to UV light so that they produce vitamin D (just as we do). One cup of these light-exposed portobello mushrooms provide 384 IUs of D, about 64 percent of a day's requirement. If you can't find these specialized mushrooms, you might want to opt for chanterelles or morels, which have a lot of naturally occurring D, or shiitakes, which are eaten regularly in Okinawa. Test-tube studies show that shiitakes ward off disease-causing microbes and kill cancer cells.

TOMATOES. If you can eat a fresh, vine-ripened tomato, you're getting the best of both worlds — life-enhancing flavor, life-extending nutrients. But don't give up on tomatoes if you can't find tasty, fresh ones. Both fresh and canned tomatoes and tomato sauce are rich in lycopene, a potent antioxidant linked to a reduced risk of cancer. The redder the tomato, the more lycopene it contains, and cooked tomatoes contain more lycopene ounce for ounce than raw and the lycopene in cooked foods is better absorbed by the body. Tomatoes are a major component of the Mediterranean-Style Diet, and a number of studies in the United States, Italy, and elsewhere have found that people who eat the most tomatoes are at lowest risk for heart disease and prostate cancer.

Herbs and Spices

Try to incorporate into your diet as often as possible.

There are no specific serving sizes; use in amounts that enhance but don't overpower the taste of your food.

Super Herbs and Spices

BASIL, CILANTRO (CORIANDER), DILL, GINGER, MINT, OREGANO, PARSLEY, ROSEMARY, AND THYME. In general, herbs and spices contain a treasure trove of compounds that fight infection and chronic diseases. I singled out these nine because they're popular in Mediterranean and/or Asian cuisine. While fresh herbs are going to have higher levels of protective compounds, for the most part, dried herbs retain enough to be helpful. The dark green herbs are rich in carotenoids, linked to a lower risk of several types of cancer. Basil, oregano, mint, parsley, rosemary, and thyme contain rosmarinic acid, which fights infection and inflammation and has been shown to fight blood clots, a major cause of strokes and heart attacks. Ginger, long known to help fight nausea, also has clot-fighting abilities and is anti-inflammatory.

Basil, cilantro, dill, mint, and parsley can be used liberally in salads — up to a quarter cup of each per four cups of other vegetables is a good ratio. Thyme, oregano, and rosemary have a stronger taste, so they stand up well to cooking (for an example, try the Braised Chicken Legs in Red Wine with Lentils, Fennel, and Kale on page 257). Add sliced ginger along with garlic to a stir-fry; chop or grate it for a sesame-oil-and-vinegar-based salad dressing or marinade. To make ginger tea, simmer a 2-inch piece of ginger, sliced into 4 pieces, in 1½ cups of water for ten minutes.

CINNAMON. Perhaps because we associate it with not-so-good-for-you treats (those giant cinnamon rolls sold in airports come to mind), cinnamon is hardly ever thought of as a healthy spice. But research shows that it has many benefits, including an ability to help combat insulin resistance. Some studies are indicating that cinnamon also reduces inflammation, can help prevent formation of AGEs (for more on these destructive compounds, see page 117), and target and eradicate cancer cells.

There are plenty of ways to get cinnamon into your diet that don't involve mammoth-size pastries. It's often used in Moroccan recipes, and it's delicious on a baked apple or in applesauce. Richard Anderson, PhD, a research chemist with the U.S. Department of Agriculture's Diet, Genomics, and Immunology Lab in Beltsville, Maryland, who has studied cinnamon, suggests soaking a cinnamon stick in hot water and drinking it like tea, or adding ground cinnamon to coffee before brewing. If you have diabetes or pre-diabetes, consuming one half teaspoon of cinnamon two times per day may help you control your blood sugar, and similar amounts may decrease AGEs and inflammation in the body. If you can't find a way to work it into the foods you're eating, you can also buy cinnamon capsules at natural food stores.

GARLIC. Garlic has an outsize reputation as a superfood—you can find claims that it prevents everything from the common cold to heart disease. So what's the truth? We do know that raw and cooked garlic is linked to a lower risk of stomach cancer and may have general immune-boosting effects. As for other benefits, according to Karin Ried, PhD, a research fellow at the University of Adelaide, Australia, who's been studying garlic, different forms of garlic have different effects. "Our review of the research found that garlic supplements—but not raw or cooked garlic—can help bring down blood pressure in people with high blood pressure," says Dr. Ried. "It's less clear whether garlic, supplements or food, reduces cholesterol; the studies are conflicting."

TURMERIC (IN CURRY POWDER OR ALONE). If you like Indian food, you're in luck. This staple of South Asian cuisine gives curry its vibrant yellow color (it's also used to color American mustard). Turmeric and one of the phyto-nutrients it contains, curcumin, are powerful anti-inflammatory agents and antioxidants. Some research shows that they both can kill cancer cells; curcumin has also been shown to clear amyloid plaque in the brains of mice, indicating that it may have potential in fighting Alzheimer's disease. A number of human studies are currently under way examining curcumin's effects on preventing and treating cancer and as a therapy for psoriasis as well as Alzheimer's.

Grains, Legumes, and Starchy Vegetables

5 to 8 servings daily, and have at least one serving at each meal, if possible

Serving = one slice of 100 percent whole grain bread; ½ cup cooked potatoes, corn, sweet potatoes, peas, or whole grains (like oatmeal, whole grain pasta, or bulgur wheat); ⅓ cup cooked legumes or brown rice

In addition to their other nutritional virtues, the grains recommended here and used in our meal plans are all whole grains, which are much higher in nutrients and fiber than refined grains. High-fiber foods are linked to lower body weight (possibly because they fill you up with fewer calories) and also fight chronic diseases in several ways, among them by lowering cholesterol. Whole grains and starchy vegetables also have a low glycemic index. The glycemic index (GI) is a 1-to-100 ranking of the extent to which a set amount of carbohydrate raises blood sugar. Low GI foods elicit the slowest and smallest rise in blood sugar; they have a GI of 55 or under. Medium GI foods fall into the 56 to 69 range and high GI foods are in the 70 to 100 range. Ideally, most of your carbs will fall into the low or medium levels, because eating this way has been linked to reduced risk for heart disease, diabetes, and obesity. The health benefits come in part because low-GI foods help keep blood sugar and insulin levels in check and keep you feeling fuller longer. One way to lower the glycemic index even further is to marinate them in or serve them tossed with a vinaigrette. Vinegar seems to encourage the flow of sugar from the blood to your cells, which helps keep blood sugar down.

Super Grains, Legumes, and Starchy Vegetables

BARLEY. The same thing that makes a mushroom barley soup so thick and hearty — a type of fiber called beta-glucan — gives barley its health benefits. Beta-glucans form a gel around food particles in your gut, slowing the absorption of sugar and starch and a corresponding slow rise in blood sugar. Preventing blood sugar spikes may help reduce your risk for pre-diabetes and type 2 diabetes, and helps control blood sugar once you have one of these conditions. Beta-glucans also slow the absorption of fat, and may actually carry fat and cholesterol out of the body before they're absorbed, thus lowering blood cholesterol. Once they're digested, the chemistry of beta-glucans seems to also reduce the body's own production of cholesterol. Think about using barley not just in soups or side dishes but also in grain salads, breads, and risottos.

BLACK RICE. In China black rice used to be called "forbidden rice" because it was reserved for emperors and noble people. Happily, it's now available to all of us — happily, because it's loaded with the same health-promoting anthocyanins as blueberries, blackberries, and red and purple grape skin. In Asia, black rice is used to make noodles, sushi, and pudding, but you can simply throw it in a pot or rice cooker and cook it like any ordinary type of rice. Many high-end markets now carry black rice, and you can find it online.

BULGUR WHEAT (CRACKED WHEAT). A staple in Middle Eastern countries, bulgur is wheat in whole grain form. What makes it different from and even healthier than whole wheat flour is its coarseness. The thicker the cut of a whole grain, the harder your body has to work to break it down, and the smaller and shorter the rise in your blood sugar will be: cooked bulgur wheat has about half the glycemic index as whole wheat bread. Bulgur is also rich in heart-protective vitamins and minerals such as vitamin E, folate, selenium, and magnesium. The most common way to eat bulgur is in tabbouleh, a Middle Eastern grain salad usually made with a slightly finer cut of bulgur and tossed with parsley, mint, lemon juice, and olive oil. Use the coarser cuts of bulgur to make pilaf (it cooks up just like rice) and combine it with beans to make veggie burgers.

STEEL-CUT OATS. Like barley, oats are a great source of beta-glucans and have all the same cholesterol-lowering effects. Opt for the steel-cut version of oats rather than flaked oats. It takes longer to cook, but this thicker and coarser cut gives it a lower glycemic index.

LEGUMES (LENTILS, CHICKPEAS, PINTO, WHITE AND BLACK BEANS). Legumes are rich in both fiber and protein. They also have other attributes, including B vitamins, magnesium, calcium, and iron, and a host of phytonutrients. Saponins, a category of phytonutrients found in legumes, reduce cholesterol levels and help fight cancer. Legumes and rice are eaten around the world in one form or another, and they make a perfect meal. It's easy to cook legumes, but if you end up buying canned, get the low-sodium or no-salt-added varieties. If those versions aren't available, be sure to rinse canned beans well before using to reduce the sodium.

SWEET POTATOES. The sweet potato is where the Okinawan Diet and the American diet cross paths: Many Okinawans eat sweet potatoes daily, and, of course, they're readily available in the United States as well, although all too often are served only on Thanksgiving. Don't just think of them as a holiday vegetable. Mash them, bake them, top them with a little maple syrup, use them in soups, but whatever you do, eat them often. Sweet potatoes contain nearly every vitamin and mineral and boast a host of phytonutrients. A medium sweet potato (about 100 calories) provides 550 percent of your daily requirement of vitamin A in the form of beta-carotene. Beta-carotene from foods (as opposed to supplements — see page 133) is linked to a lower risk of cancer and heart disease.

Milk/Soy Milk Products

2 to 3 servings daily

Serving = 1 cup milk or calcium-fortified soy milk; ¾ cup plain yogurt

I recommend nonfat and 1% milk and yogurt throughout this plan because milk is the main source of calcium in the American diet and these foods are also rich in magnesium and potassium. These fat-free and very low fat products ensure you don't overdo calories or saturated fat. They're also associated with a decreased risk of osteoporosis and colon cancer. I'm stopping short of calling them superfoods because there is evidence that milk may slightly raise the risk of prostate cancer. Of course, anyone worried about this can switch to calcium-enriched soy milk, a perfect substitute.

High-Protein Foods

5 to 8 servings daily

Serving = 1 ounce fatty fish or dark meat poultry; 1½ ounces white fish or light meat poultry; 60 calories tofu, which works out to 1½ to 3½ ounces, depending on the type, so check labels; 1 to 1½ ounces tempeh (same thing — it varies); ⅔ cup legumes

Your protein strategy: Have any of the fatty fish listed on the following page three times a week. Try to get in at least 12 ounces weekly, more if you like fish. Your other high-protein staples should be skinless poultry, eggs, egg whites, egg white products, and soy (tofu, tempeh, edamame). Though other legumes (such as black beans, pinto beans, and white beans) don't have as complete a protein profile as soy, it's fine to use them as your protein source for one meal daily. Limit your intake of red meat to no more than three times a month or less. This may seem Draconian if you're used to eating meat several times a week, but my reasoning comes by way of many studies showing that frequently eating red meat raises the risk for colon cancer and increases the risk for heart disease. Processed meats such as hot dogs, bacon, pepperoni, and sausages, all high in saturated fat, are particularly unhealthful. Avoid them or eat them only occasionally.

Super High-Protein Foods

FATTY FISH (WILD-CAUGHT SALMON, TROUT, SARDINES). In general, fish is a healthy protein choice, but these fish are the top of the line. Not only are they richer in healthy omega-3 fatty acids (see page 107) than other types of fish, but they are also lower in mercury and other pollutants than many of the fish in the seafood case. The fish supply, including some fish farmed in other countries and imported, has become very contaminated, and I recom-

---

Is Soy Safe?

The messages are conflicting. On the one hand soy is referred to as a superfood. On the other hand, some say it might be a trigger for breast cancer. Which is true? There's no doubt that soy is a healthy source of protein, and a good substitute for meat. But soy also contains phytoestrogens, weak forms of the body's natural hormone, and that has raised some concerns. About 70 percent of breast cancers are estrogen positive, meaning that the hormone causes cancerous cells to grow. It could be that phytoestrogens simply add to your estrogen load, encouraging cells to become cancerous.

Yet there is some other thinking on the topic. It may be that phytoestrogens compete with real estrogen for landing sites on breast and other cells, and because they're much weaker cancer-promoters than estrogen, actually help protect you from cancer. Soy actually does seem to have a protective effect against breast cancer when it's consumed early in life. However, whether soy consumed in high amounts confers that same protective effect—or, conversely, a harmful effect—in adult women is still unknown.

The American Institute for Cancer Research recommends limiting soy to two to three servings a day. If you're undergoing any anti-estrogen treatments (such as tamoxifen), it's recommended that you avoid soy altogether. Most important, avoid high-dose isoflavone supplements (isoflavones are an active ingredient in soy) if you're receiving treatment for breast cancer—and even if you're not. There's no evidence showing that they have health benefits.

mend that you be careful (visit the Monterey Bay Aquarium's Seafood Watch website to keep updated on the safest fish and those that are sustainably fished: www.montereybayaquarium.org/cr/seafoodwatch.aspx).

Fish in general confers numerous health benefits. Regular fish consumption has been linked to a lower risk of dementia, and a Harvard University study tracking thousands of men found that those eating fish at least once a week were only half as likely to experience sudden cardiac death as those who ate no fish. In that study, all types of fish were beneficial, but fatty fish has the added benefit of having high levels of omega-3s. And these fish oils may not be the only heart-protective factor. Fatty fish are also low in saturated fat, and many contain vitamin D.

SOY (TOFU, TEMPEH, EDAMAME). As many people move away from red meat, they're moving more toward soy, and with good reason. Soy is a good source of high-quality protein and unsaturated fat (both tempeh and edamame are also fiber rich) and has been shown to lower blood cholesterol. It may reduce the risk of certain cancers, although this is still uncertain (see "Is Soy Safe?" at left). One of the beauties of soy is that it comes in so many forms. Edamame are young green soybeans available in the frozen section of the supermarket (both shelled and in the pod). You can use them in stir-fries and soups and as a snack. Tempeh is made from cooking mature soybeans and adding a mold culture (cheese is made that way, too); grains are often also added. It has a pleasant, nutty taste and a satisfying chewy consistency. Tempeh works well in hot and cold foods and makes a great sandwich. Tofu is made from soy milk and comes in various consistencies. Firm tofu is great marinated and baked or in stir-fries; soft, silken tofu works nicely in soups (it's often added to miso soup) or made into scrambles. There are also a lot of soy-based prepared foods on the market that are both healthy and convenient. Gardein, for example, makes a whole line of soy products that mimic chicken and beef.

EGG WHITES. The white of an egg is the perfect protein, with ideal levels of amino acids (the building blocks of protein). Whole eggs, of course, are very nutritious, too, but one large egg contains some saturated fat (1.5 g) and lots of cholesterol (211 mg) — almost all of it contained in the yolk. For most people cholesterol in food doesn't raise blood cholesterol. But if you're one of the few for whom it does cause a problem (you'd know it if you lowered your dietary cholesterol and your lab values improved), egg whites are a better choice than whole eggs. Even if you don't have high cholesterol, if you're eating a lot of eggs it's a good idea to alternate egg whites and whole eggs to keep your saturated fat intake low. Also consider using an egg white product such as Better'n Eggs. The ready-to-use egg whites are convenient, they contain added vitamins and minerals, and they're pasteurized so there's no risk of salmonella.

Nuts, Nut Butters, and Seeds

1–2 servings daily

Serving = ½ ounce, about 2 tablespoons nuts or 1 tablespoon nut butter. All nuts are healthful because they have great fat profiles and contain phytonutrients, but the ones below are standouts.

Super Nuts and Seeds

ALMONDS. Packed with a laundry list of nutrients, phytonutrients, and healthy fats, *unsalted* almonds not only helped lower LDL cholesterol in the Portfolio Diet but were largely responsible for reducing blood pressure. Toss almonds into salads, eat them as a snack, add sliced ones to chicken or fish dishes, but use restraint. They're healthy, but, like all nuts, still high in calories: an ounce has 170.

FLAXSEED. Flaxseed and flaxseed oil are the richest source of plant-based omega-3s and therefore offer all the benefits of these essential fatty acids. Flaxseed is also a good source of fiber (although flaxseed oil is not), and it contains phytoestrogens — the type of phytoestrogen in flaxseed is called lignan — so the same question that dogs soy (see "Is Soy Safe?," page 102) dogs flaxseed as well. In an attempt to answer that question, scientists at the German Cancer Research Center in Heidelberg reviewed the research on lignans and breast cancer and concluded that postmenopausal women taking in higher levels of lignans have about a 15 percent lower risk of developing breast cancer, and that studies show no effect either way on premenopausal women's risk.

There are a few things to keep in mind about flaxseed. You need to grind them to get all their benefits; your body won't break down whole ones. Because omega-3s oxidize (go rancid) quickly, it's best to buy whole flaxseeds, keep them refrigerated, then grind them in a coffee or spice grinder, a food processor, or high-quality blender. Grind in small batches (a week's worth of the flaxseed called for in the 20 Years Younger Diet is about ½ cup). Place the ground flaxseed in an airtight container or plastic bag and store them in the refrigerator. You can sprinkle ground flaxseed on cereal, add to muffin, cookie, and bread recipes, and stir into yogurt and smoothies. Add flaxseed oil to sauces and salad dressings.

WALNUTS. Walnuts are a powerhouse of nutrients and a good vegetarian source of omega-3 fatty acids. They're not quite as good as the type of omega-3s in fish, but your body can convert a portion of them into the more advantageous kind. Walnuts are also high in vitamin E, melatonin, and ellagic acid (see berries), and the fat in the walnuts may make it even easier for your body to absorb these compounds. One more reason walnuts belong in the superfood category: In conjunction with an overall healthy diet, they not only help lower LDL (bad) cholesterol levels but bring down the most artery-clogging type of cholesterol, called dense LDL.

Fats

4 to 7 servings daily

Serving = 1 teaspoon of oil, mayonnaise, or healthy spread (made without partially hydrogenated oil); 1 tablespoon light mayonnaise, light healthy spread, or regular salad dressing; 2 tablespoons light salad dressing; ⅕ of a Haas avocado

NOTE: Nuts and nut butter can also be used as fats, so if you want more nuts than your allotted serving (see Nuts, Nut Butters, and Seeds above), go ahead — just count them as a fat serving. One tablespoon of nuts or 1½ teaspoons of nut butter is a fat serving.

Superfats

Fats are a confusing issue, so let's talk about not just superfats but your approach to fats in general. Long vilified, fats are actually essential to health and longevity, but it's important to distinguish the healthy ones from the ones that can do damage. There are two fats you need to watch: saturated and trans fats, both of which raise blood cholesterol levels. Limit saturated fat (found in animal foods) as much as possible and try to avoid trans fats (found in hydrogenated oils) completely.

One of the fats you do want in your diet is monounsaturated fat, the primary type of fat in olive oil. If you think you like olive oil, get this: Greeks currently take in an average of 100 cups of olive oil per year. All that oil contributes to longevity in a few ways. Among them: Anti-inflammatory compounds in olive oil called polyphenols help prevent cardiovascular disease and cancer. The monounsaturated fat in olive oil's makeup — about 70 percent of its total fat — lowers levels of LDL (bad) cholesterol and helps prevent its oxidation. LDL oxidation leads to clogging and hardening of the arteries. The monounsaturated fatty acids in olive oil have also been linked to a reduction of body fat storage and a higher fat-burning rate in the five hours after having an olive oil–rich meal.

As wonderful as olive oil is, there may be times when you want a neutral-tasting oil. That's where canola oil comes in. It also has a stellar nutrition profile — it's lower in saturated fat than most other oils, has about the same level of monounsaturated fat as olive oil, and is a rich source of ALA, plant omega-3s, which I'll tell you more about shortly. Studies show that using canola oil on a regular basis helps reduce LDL (bad) cholesterol. Others show that it slightly raises HDL (good) cholesterol.

Polyunsaturated fats, to varying degree, are also beneficial. Polyunsaturated fat is the dominant fat in most other vegetable oils. Among polyunsaturated oils are soybean oil, corn oil, and sunflower oil. These contain fatty acids known as omega-6s, which are the building blocks of cell membranes. While they don't raise blood cholesterol, consumed in excess, omega-6s can cause inflammation and "thicken" the blood, making it more likely to form blood clots. That can lead to heart attacks and stroke, so you need to be cautious about overconsuming these particular polyunsaturates.

In a different category altogether is the type of polyunsaturated fat with the most anti-aging and overall health benefits: omega-3 fatty acids, found in fish oils and in some plant foods. They're linked to a reduced risk of heart disease, cancer, and diabetes and are anti-inflammatory and integral to healthy brain function, and may even help ease depression. Some studies show that people with higher-than-average levels of omega-3s in their blood have a lower risk of dementia.

Omega-6 fatty acids compete with omega-3s for entry into cell membranes, the reason you want to keep the two in balance. We were designed to eat omega-3s and omega-6s in equal amounts, according to Artemis Simopoulos, MD, director of the Center for Genetics, Nutrition, and Health in Washington, D.C., who's researched dietary fats extensively. "During our evolution, nearly all foods contained omega-3 fatty acids. But now, very few foods are good sources," says Dr. Simopoulos. "For instance, game animals used to graze on grass and other wild plants, which made their meat rich in omega-3s; now cattle eat corn and other feed, which results in meat virtually devoid of omega-3s." Instead of the 1:1 omega-6 to omega-3 ratio we were designed for, the typical American diet has a 16:1 ratio. By contrast, the traditional Greek diet has a ratio between 1:1 and 1:2, and the Japanese ratio is about 4:1.

The most potent types of omega-3s are those found in fish: eicosopentaenoic acid (EPA) and docosahexaenoic acid (DHA). However, alpha-linolenic acid (ALA), prevalent in plant foods, is still effective and important to include in your diet. Dr. Simopoulos recommends taking in 2,000 mg of ALA daily (slightly higher than that recommended by the Institute of Medicine), and at least 650 mg of EPA and DHA combined. The best way to reach that goal is to eat at least one omega-3-rich food daily. "And just to ensure you're getting enough omega-3s, take a daily supplement of 1,000 milligrams," advises Dr. Simopoulos.

Your Good Fat Guide

OKAY, BUT ONLY IN MODERATION

Foods high in omega-6s: corn oil, sunflower oil, safflower oil, soybean oil, peanut oil, and all the foods made from these oils, such as many salad dressings, sauces, and fried foods.

VERY GOOD

Foods high in plant-based omega-3, alpha-linolenic acid (ALA): flaxseed, flaxseed oil, walnuts, omega-3-enriched foods such as some eggs.

EXCELLENT

Foods high in monounsaturated fat: olive oil, canola oil, almonds, cashews, avocados. Also: foods high in EPA and DHA: fatty fish including bluefish, mackerel, trout, salmon, and sardines (these are also low in mercury, which, in excess, can cause a number of health issues including damaged nerves).

Healthy Treats

Between 150 and 250 calories daily (see page 91 to see the amount that corresponds to your overall calorie level)

Serving sizes vary, so check labels to find the appropriate portion for your particular treat calorie limit.

Your sweets and treats strategy: We have a natural predilection for foods that are sweet, yet it's also our Achilles' heel. Too many sweets, of course, add up to too many calories, and they're typically empty calories — that is, generally unaccompanied by any vitamins, minerals, or fiber. The one supertreat on this list — chocolate — compensates by providing a healthy dose of antioxidants. Two other treats—poached or baked apples or pears and fruit topped with slightly sweetened yogurt or tossed with a mix of citrus juice and honey—are good choices, too. Eat them in moderation to satisfy your sweet tooth without overindulging.

Supertreats

Cocoa powder and dark chocolate (over 50 percent cacao). Sometimes you luck out and a food that you really love is also good for you. That's the case with cocoa and dark chocolate; their health benefits stem from compounds called flavanols, antioxidants that also stimulate your body to produce nitric oxide, which opens up arteries, reducing blood pressure. Nitric oxide also discourages plaque formation in the arteries, another way it protects the heart. Scientists became clued in to cocoa's blood-pressure-lowering effects when they found that a Panamanian Indian tribe with a high cocoa consumption had virtually none of the age-related rise in blood pressure and kidney disease (a consequence of high blood pressure) found in most societies. Their cardiovascular death rates were also an astonishingly low 9 per 100,000 people compared to 83 per 100,000 in the rest of Pan-America. But when members of the tribe moved out of their villages and into urban Panama City, they ate much less cocoa and their heart disease rates shot up to those in the rest of the country.

Pure unsweetened cocoa is richest in flavanols, followed by dark chocolate (at least 50 percent cacao or, as it's sometimes referred to, cocoa). Milk chocolate usually doesn't have too many flavanols. The only real drawback to dark chocolate is that at 140 calories per ounce, it's easy to rack up a lot of calories if you don't carefully monitor your portion sizes. (Chocolate is also high in saturated fat, but it's a saturated fat called stearic acid, which doesn't raise LDL cholesterol and may lower blood pressure.) You can be a little more liberal with unsweetened cocoa: It only has 12 calories per tablespoon.

DON'T GET SWEET ON SUGAR SUBSTITUTES

Because maintaining a healthy weight can be critical to longevity, it might seem reasonable to use artificial sweeteners to help control calories. After all, you save 16 calories for each teaspoon of sugar, honey, fruit juice sweetener, or other calorie-containing sweetener that you replace with an artificial one. But it isn't at all clear whether making the swap actually saves you calories over the long haul. In fact, some studies show that consuming sugar substitutes may actually cause weight *gain*. The San Antonio Heart study, for instance, tracked people who began the study with a similar body mass index (BMI; see page 122 for an explanation). Seven to eight years later, the researchers found that those people who consumed the most artificial sweetener had a BMI one point higher than those participants who consumed very few artificially sweetened foods.

One explanation may be that sugar substitutes don't satisfy in the same way that real sweeteners do. Sure, a diet soda tastes sweet and may gratify a sweet craving, but that's not the only way your body reads satisfaction; it also keeps track of calories, and it knows when you're trying to fake it out. Plus, artificial sweeteners like sucralose (brand name Splenda), aspartame (Nutrasweet), acesulfame K (Sunett), and saccharin (Sweet'N Low) tend to be incredibly sweet — sweeter than a natural sweetener. That can make you become accustomed to very sweet foods and drinks so that you crave cookies, cakes, and other high-calorie foods.

There is, too, the issue of safety. To my mind, we just don't know enough, even if artificial sweeteners are approved by the FDA. Here's what I recommend: If you drink traditional types of soda to excess and using artificial sweeteners helps you wean yourself off all that sugar, then it may be worthwhile to use them for a short time. But beyond that, you don't need them. Work toward keeping your intake of sweet foods moderate, and when you do eat sweets, go for the real thing.

WHAT SHOULD YOU DRINK?

Beverages often get treated as an afterthought, but they're an important part of a healthy diet. My suggestion: Drink at least 6 eight-ounce cups of water daily, and no more than about 4 cups of coffee or tea (caffeine tolerance is very individual; if you're jittery or not sleeping well, these limits may be too high for you). Have as much herbal tea as you like. Wine, like any alcohol, is optional. If you do drink alcohol (see page 113), have no more than one drink daily if you're a woman; no more than two drinks if you're a man. Typical serving sizes are 8 ounces water; 8 ounces tea or coffee; 5 ounces wine; 12 ounces beer; 1½ ounces hard liquor. Here are some specifics about the beverages you may include in the 20 Years Younger Diet.

Plain water, sparkling water, or water with a splash of juice. The best thing you can drink is water, no question. It has no calories, and it helps keep every process in your body running smoothly. If you're dehydrated you're not going to get the most out of your workout — dehydration lowers your endurance. Water is what your body was designed to drink.

I find that people usually fall into two camps: those who love drinking water all day and those who find water utterly boring and really have to struggle to get in 6 cups a day. For those of you who need a little flavor, sparkling water with juice is the perfect solution, especially if you're weaning yourself off soda. Simply add a tablespoon or two of your favorite juice (cranberry, pomegranate, and mango are all good choices) to a glass of sparkling water, stir, and sip.

Coffee. Coffee is what you might call a mixed bag. On the one hand, some research shows that people who drink a lot of coffee (5 to 7 cups daily) have a substantially lower risk of diabetes. This is likely due to compounds in coffee called chlorogenic acids, which help slow the rise in blood sugar. (Decaf may also lower the risk of diabetes.) Chlorogenic acids are also strong antioxidants that may protect against estrogen-related cancers. These antioxidants may be the reason that coffee drinkers have a lower risk for developing dementia, Parkinson's disease, and Alzheimer's, too.

Yet coffee also has its drawbacks. It may exacerbate ovarian cysts, and its effects on the heart are still an open question. And coffee, of course, can interfere with sleep; anything that keeps you from being well rested isn't doing you any favors. To be on the safe side, follow the guidelines stated earlier — no more than 4 cups of coffee daily — to keep your coffee intake moderate and bear in mind that decaffeinated coffee can confer the same benefits as caffeinated without the big buzz.

Tea. Could tea be one of the reasons Okinawans live so long? Perhaps. It certainly has many healthful qualities. In general, tea drinkers have a lower risk of stroke and heart disease. Tea is also linked to a lower risk of Alzheimer's and Parkinson's diseases. In one study, people who drank two or more cups of black tea daily were 60 percent less likely to develop Parkinson's. Tea drinkers are also at reduced risk for lung and colon cancers.

The key anti-aging ingredients in tea are phytonutrients called catechins. Green tea and black tea contain different types of catechins, but both types are antioxidants and anti-inflammatory agents, which help prevent clogged arteries and neutralize cancer-causing agents. Because the caffeine content of tea is one-third to half that of coffee, it's safer for the heart and less likely to interfere with sleep. Nonetheless, pay attention to how you feel and cap your intake if you feel jittery.

Wine. Both red and white wine are consumed in moderation, and usually with meals, throughout the Mediterranean. Wine drinkers have a reduced risk of heart disease and death from any cause. This seems to be due to both the alcohol itself and the phytonutrients in wine, including anthocyanins, phenolic acids, and a polyphenol called resveratrol (see grapes on page 93). Some scientists believe resveratrol shows promise for the prevention of many age-related conditions, including Parkinson's and Alzheimer's diseases, inflammation, diabetes, and cardiovascular disease.

Remember that the Mediterranean people get health benefits from drinking *moderately*. Excessive drinking reverses the rewards of wine (see "Can Alcohol Help You Live Longer — Or Shorten Your Life?" opposite).

Can Alcohol Help You Live Longer — Or Shorten Your Life?

In general, research studies show that one to two drinks for women and two to up to four drinks for men is beneficial, conferring a 30 percent lower risk of dying of heart disease and a 20 percent reduction of dying from any cause. Yet not everyone is so sure alcohol's benefits outweigh its risks. Some cite the fact that even moderate drinking is linked to an increased risk of several types of cancer, including cancer of the breast, liver, and colon. And there's no doubt that heavy and binge drinking increases the risk of cancer, damages the heart, and causes a whole host of other health problems. After a few glasses, the law of diminishing returns takes hold and alcohol becomes harmful, not helpful.

It's my opinion that you can get most of the same heart-healthy benefits from exercise, certain foods, and even doses of baby aspirin (check with your physician) that you can get from alcohol without the risk of cancer and the liver disease cirrhosis. Those options don't have the calories of alcohol either. One way red wine is thought to lower risks to the heart is by thinning the blood. Exercise does that, and so does aspirin. Wine is also being touted for its resveratrol content, but grapes offer resveratrol (with the added bonus of fiber, too). I'm not a teetotaler, but I do keep in mind that alcohol can disrupt a healthy lifestyle. When you imbibe, you may lose inhibitions and tend to eat less cautiously, and you're going to be less likely to exercise If you've been drinking or wake up fuzzy from a night of margaritas.

If you've had a history or family history of any of the cancers connected to alcohol (go to www.cancer.org for more information on which cancers are linked to alcohol use), you'll especially want to keep drinking to a minimum. My recommendation is the same as the American Cancer Society's: limit intake to one to two drinks a day for men and one drink a day for women—a happy medium that may allow you to get some of the heart-protective perks without the cancer risk.

Remember that the health benefits of wine top out after a glass or two. And while moderate drinking may protect the heart, excessive drinking can damage it. Err on the side of limiting your consumption of alcohol.

WHAT *NOT* TO EAT: FOODS THAT AGE YOU

Just as certain foods slow down the aging process, others can speed it up, and you need look no further than the typical American diet: burgers, fries, white bread, sodas, candy, doughnuts, giant muffins, sweetened coffee drinks, buffalo wings, potato chips.

These foods are rife with substances that promote inflammation and oxidation, raise blood pressure and cholesterol levels, and damage DNA. In that way, they raise your risk for just about every chronic disease. Here are the killer compounds that you need to either avoid or limit:

Trans Fats

The main source of this type of fat is partially hydrogenated oil. This is an oil, such as soybean, put through a chemical process that solidifies it into margarine or shortening. These fats were at one time considered a healthier alternative to lard and butter, which are high in saturated fat. But now we know that trans fat is the most dangerous fat around. It promotes inflammation and the storage of intra-abdominal fat, and it raises LDL (bad) cholesterol while lowering HDL, the good kind.

YOUR STRATEGY: Always check the ingredient list for "partially hydrogenated oil." Often you'll find that foods containing this oil still state 0 g of trans fat on the nutrition label. That's because a labeling loophole allows for a "0" if a product has under 0.5 grams of trans (or any other type of) fat. Taking in even one or two grams of this fat is considered too much, so you can see how eating only a few servings that contain just under half a gram can quickly add up. So put back on the shelf any product containing partially hydrogenated oil. At restaurants, skip pies—the crusts may be made with shortening—and pass on fried and heavily breaded foods. If you have a recipe that calls for shortening or margarine, look for the kinds that are made without any partially hydrogenated oils, such as the Bestlife buttery spread and the new Bestlife buttery baking sticks.

Saturated Fat

This fat lurks mainly (though not only) in foods of animal origin such as red meat, bacon, chicken skin, whole and 2% milk, and cream. Like trans fats, saturated fat promotes inflammation, especially if you're overweight. It lodges in the fat cells and turns them into little inflammation factories, and this can ultimately lead to insulin resistance, heart disease, diabetes, and cancer.

If you need some numbers as guideposts, most people can get away with just under 10 percent of calories from saturated fat. The Okinawan and Mediterranean-Style Diets go a little lower — 7 percent. This is also the amount recommended if you have heart disease. On a 1,500 calorie-per-day diet, 10 percent is 15 g saturated fat; on a 1,700-calorie diet, it's 17 g.

YOUR STRATEGY: You can't avoid this fat, as even healthy foods such as nuts, olive oil, and canola oil contain some saturated fat. But if you avoid the other sources mentioned above, you'll automatically significantly reduce your saturated fat intake. Food labels are required to list the saturated fat content, so when buying any type of food — frozen foods, cheese, crackers, cereal, desserts — always compare labels and pick the items lowest in saturated fat.

Sodium

While a little sodium is critical to our health and survival — among other things it helps regulate the heartbeat and blood volume and is necessary for proper nerve function — too much can age us in a number of ways. A high-sodium diet contributes to high blood pressure in many people, and high blood pressure is the cause of 62 percent of stroke cases and 49 percent of heart disease cases (it also contributes to kidney disease and stomach cancer). Health organizations have been recommending that Americans cap sodium levels at 2,300 mg daily and those with high blood pressure take in no more than 1,500 mg. But now that the majority of Americans have high blood pressure or are considered sodium-sensitive, recent government guidelines extend the 1,500 mg daily upper limit for people who are fifty-one or older, African Americans of any age, and people who have diabetes or chronic kidney disease. My meal plan tops out at 2,300 mg sodium per day; any lower is very difficult to attain if you eat out at all. If you need to drop down to 1,500, adjust the plan by using reduced-sodium bread and cheese and choosing the lowest-sodium foods you can find. You might also eliminate the little bit of salt in 20 Years Younger recipes.

YOUR STRATEGY: Buy the lowest sodium foods you can in every category. Do this by comparing food labels when you shop — pretty soon you'll have a repertoire of staples and won't have to be so vigilant. Because you never know how much sodium's been added to restaurant food, assume the worst. On days that you eat out, make sure the meals you eat at home are very low in sodium (aim for no more than 400 mg).

To meet the 2,300 mg sodium limit, the menus beginning on page 225 are very light in salt; perhaps lighter than you're used to. If you're finding it a tough adjustment, take out the salt shaker and sprinkle just a few crystals on the food on your plate. This will give you a much stronger hit of saltiness than if you'd poured a lot more salt into the food as it was being prepared.

Sugar

Americans are eating way too much sugar, and not just white table sugar, but high-fructose corn syrup, honey, fruit juice sweetener, and maple, brown rice, and agave syrups, too. Much of this sugar is coming from sodas and other sugary drinks, which contain about 10 teaspoons of sugar per 12 ounces (and many people are buying 16- and 24-ounce servings). Here's the problem with all that sugar: The nutritionally empty calories promote obesity, wreak havoc on the system of anyone whose blood sugar is even a little high, and cause the formation of age-promoting AGE compounds (see the following section).

YOUR STRATEGY: While the naturally occurring sugar found in fruits and milk is fine, limit added sugar (the stuff you sweeten your coffee with and the sugar found in sweet beverages, desserts, candy, and unexpected places such as salad dressing and barbecue sauce) to no more than 8 percent of your total calories. That's 30 g of added sugar on a 1,500-calorie-per-day diet; 34 g on a 1,700-calorie diet, and 40 g on a 2,000-calorie diet. Glance at the sugar column on the nutrition label and see how quickly you can hit your limit. There are 33 g of sugar in a 12-ounce soda; 25 g in a roll of Life Savers. I'd skip sodas and sugary beverages completely — not only are they excessively high in sugar, but your body barely notices those calories because liquid calories don't fill you up nearly as well as calories in solid food.

Unfortunately, nutrition labels don't distinguish added sugar from naturally occurring, so you have to use the ingredient list to figure it out. If there's no fruit or dairy in the ingredient list, then all or nearly all the sugar is added. For something like ice cream or flavored yogurt, it's impossible to tell what percent of sugar is from the milk and what's coming from added sugar, but figure it's at least half and half.

ANTI-AGE-ING COOKING

The way you prepare a food affects its health properties. Add a little oil to a salad or lightly sauté vegetables in oil and you'll absorb a lot more carotenoids because they tend to cling to fat particles. Steamed or microwaved vegetables tend to retain more vitamin C and other nutrients than fried or roasted; and the longer a vegetable is cooked, the fewer nutrients it retains.

Cooking meat, poultry, and fish at very high heat (frying, grilling, and broiling) creates heterocyclic amines (HCAs), which are known to promote cancer. Other carcinogens produced by grilling are polycyclic aromatic hydrocarbons (PAHs); they're formed when fat drips out of the meat (as well as vegetables and even bread rubbed with oil) and comes back as smoke that is absorbed by the food.

Though nutrition experts have been sounding the alarm about HCAs and PAHs for years now, there's another dangerous side effect to high-temperature cooking that's just starting to show up on the radar: AGEs. Aptly named, these "advanced glycation end products" speed up the aging process. We form AGEs in our bodies as well as consume them; they're contained in many foods. When AGEs hit a critical mass they can cause inflammation, clogged arteries, cataracts, wrinkles and sagging skin, and kidney and nervous system damage. AGEs are formed in the body when sugars, such as blood glucose, combine with amino acids, the building blocks of proteins and other substances. High blood sugar is a major trigger of AGE formation because it means there's a lot more sugar available to combine with amino acids. "The higher your blood sugar, the more AGEs you'll form," says Jaime Uribarri, MD, professor of medicine, Mount Sinai School of Medicine in New York City. A nephrologist (kidney doctor), Dr. Uribarri has been researching the effects of AGEs on kidney disease.

While eating sugar doesn't necessarily make you more susceptible to AGE damage (unless you gain so much weight from your sweet diet that you develop high blood sugar), certain foods that contain high levels of AGEs do. Fresh fruits and vegetables, bread, and grains are lowest in AGEs, while foods of animal origin, such as meat, poultry, fish, and cheese are highest, particularly when they're cooked at high heat. "AGE levels rise when foods are cooked, and the higher the cooking temperature, the more AGEs produced," says Dr. Uribarri. "Grilling, broiling, roasting, searing, and frying are the worst offenders."

For instance, AGEs in beef go up ninefold when you broil it; twelvefold when stir-fried. But use a lower temperature cooking method such as microwaving or stewing, and AGE levels only triple. Sautéed tofu has six times the AGEs of raw, but boiled tofu has only 20 percent more. Potatoes, like most fruits and vegetables, are very low in AGEs to begin with, but turn them into french fries and levels spike a staggering eighty-nine-fold. So far, of all the foods Dr. Uribarri and his colleagues have analyzed, fried bacon is the worst offender. The runner-up is roasted chicken skin (another good reason, besides lowering the fat content of your meal, to remove the skin from poultry).

People who regularly consume a high AGE diet have significantly higher levels of AGEs in their blood. But when they're placed on a low AGE diet, not only do blood levels of AGEs fall — by about 30 percent — but more important, so do markers of disease risk, such as inflammation and oxidative stress. The menus starting on page 225 are good examples of how to lower your intake of AGEs. Most of the meat, poultry, and fish are poached, steamed, or stewed. Many of those foods are marinated, too: Cooking with a sauce containing vinegar or lemon juice tends to reduce AGE formation during heating, another good way to reduce your risk.

HOW LOW CAN YOU GO: THE SCIENCE OF CALORIE RESTRICTION

One of the hottest topics among anti-aging researchers is calorie restriction, consuming an exceptionally low number of calories as a strategy for life extension. The 20 Years Younger Diet is not a calorie restriction diet along the same lines as those being researched right now (though it can help you lower your calorie intake enough to lose weight). But I thought you might be interested to know a little about it. It's definitely a subject you'll be hearing more about in the future.

The connection between calorie restriction and longevity was first made in the 1930s when studies showed that in mice, cutting calories by 30 to 50 percent but keeping their diet nutritious extended their life span by 50 percent. Calorie restriction has even been shown to double the life span of some insects. And now major research institutions such as the National Institute on Aging are investigating whether it will work on humans—and whether it's even practical. Some people aren't waiting for the results; the Calorie Restriction (CR) Society International, an organization devoted to the practice, has upwards of 4,000 members.

How It Works

Why would significantly restricting calories extend life—and even make you healthier? One reason is that it lowers body fat and, as you might remember from chapter 1, excess body fat is linked to inflammation and insulin resistance, among other harbingers of disease. Also, when you're not getting quite enough calories, your body responds by slowing down its metabolism. In this context, it's important to understand that "metabolism" doesn't just refer to the rate at which your body burns calories. Metabolism also refers to other chemical reactions in your body, including cell division. When the metabolism slows, the body shifts its focus from cell growth and reproduction to repair and maintenance of tissues, which slows down the aging process.

Calorie restriction has been found to slow down both "primary aging," the damage done to cells from things like free radicals, and "secondary aging," the development of diseases such as cancer, says Pennington Biomedical Research Center's Donald Williamson, PhD. Pennington is one of the three research centers in the country carrying out the largest human calorie restriction study. It's called CALERIE and is funded by the National Institute on Aging. When researchers measure cellular biomarkers of aging (such as telomere length and responsiveness of the immune system) in calorie-deprived rats, 90 percent of the biomarkers stay at youthful levels. Calorie-restricted rats and mice also postpone, or don't ever get, cancer and diabetes.

In animal studies, calorie restriction starts in what's roughly the equivalent of the late teenage years in humans. "Based on this research, the ideal age to start calorie restriction would be age twenty," says Dr. Williamson. "But there's some evidence — still iffy — that it could do you some good starting later, at age forty or even fifty." The difference would be that you'd likely get secondary aging benefits — that is, a lower risk of life-threatening disease — rather than much deterrence of primary aging.

Is It Worth It?

I was once talking to a friend about calorie restriction when he said, "I'm not sure if it helps you live longer or it just feels that way." I get his point. It's hard to live on such a low-calorie diet. What's more, it will take decades to know whether calorie restriction can extend human life without harmful effects because studies such as CALERIE are only just getting started. But we may have some clues because diet surveys were conducted in Okinawa beginning in 1949 and repeated at various intervals afterward. "Based on the surveys, it looks like the older generation in Okinawa has been taking in fewer calories than needed since they were in their twenties," says Okinawa International University's Dr. Willcox. Perhaps that's one reason why the Okinawans, who've stayed slender all their lives, have managed to live so long. It's also interesting to note that when researchers tested the blood of Okinawans in their seventies to measure the hormone DHEA, their levels were significantly higher than those of Americans of the same age. Because DHEA is known to diminish with age, higher levels are indicative of a more youthful biology. (Calorie-restricted animals also have higher DHEA levels.)

The CALERIE studies are already showing that calorie restriction reduces — no surprise — obesity, and that it also lowers inflammation and insulin sensitivity. It improves a number of other heart disease risk factors as well: LDL cholesterol, blood pressure, and heart rate go down, and the blood becomes less likely to clot. But doesn't plain old diet and exercise accomplish all this? Yes, but based on animal studies, a calorie restriction diet is poised to do more. One reason is that calorie restriction isn't just any old weight-loss diet; it's an incredibly nutritious one, in which every bite (and you don't get many!) counts. High levels of vitamins, minerals, and phytonutrients work in tandem with the slowing of the metabolism to stave off aging as long as possible. Another way calorie restriction differs from a typical weight-loss diet is that even after you lose excess weight, you continue restricting — for life — taking in about 20 to 25 percent less than your daily energy needs *before* you began the calorie restriction. (So if you maintained your weight at 2,000 calories before you started restricting calories, then you'd still eat 20 to 25 percent less — 1,500 to 1,600 calories per day — even after you've lost weight.)

Now here's where, to my exercise physiologist mind, it gets complicated. Calorie restriction's anti-aging effects hinge largely on slowing down metabolism. Exercise does just the opposite; it speeds it up. Dr. Williamson, though, puts it in perspective. "Exercise does play an important anti-aging role. It helps you maintain the fat loss you've achieved through calorie restriction; that's critical because excess body fat hastens aging. And exercise has its own effects on aging, such as reducing inflammation and reducing chronic disease risk," he says. "But based on lab animal research, exercise alone doesn't extend life; you have to add caloric restriction to the mix to get the deep cuts in primary aging."

The big question is, how low into calorie restriction can most people go? If you're eating 2,000 calories a day now, a 20 to 25 percent restriction will translate into about 400 to 500 fewer calories a day (a level you can meet by following the lowest calorie plan on the 20 Years Younger Diet). You don't have to become rail thin to get the benefits, and no one should dip below a body mass index of 18.5. (Your body mass index is a measure of your weight in relation to your height. You can calculate yours at 20YearsYounger.com.) And there are some other caveats, says Dr. Williamson. Calorie restriction isn't for anyone younger than age twenty (it might interfere with growth and development) or older than sixty-five, because of the risk of losing muscle and bone along with body fat. Plus, there's evidence that carrying a little more weight is protective in your older years.

We have a lot more to learn before we can make any practical recommendations about calorie restriction. There's currently a lot of time and money being spent on the research, but it's difficult to know how much of the population will be willing or able to drop their calories to a minimum in order to extend their lives. "There's no glossing over it — it's hard work," says Dr. Williamson. It may be that you don't even need to drop calories very low to extend your life. We already know that a healthy diet coupled with a vigorous exercise regimen can go a long way toward increasing your life span. Check my website for updates on calorie restriction.

A REASONABLE APPROACH TO SUPPLEMENTS

By Diane L. McKay, PhD

The 20 Years Younger Diet is designed to bolster your intake of fruits, vegetables and whole grains, the foods so many people neglect. Without adequate intake of these foods, you're certain to miss out on some of the nutrients you need to keep aging at bay. But even if you're bucking the trend and actually eating a healthful diet, there's still a case to be made for taking supplements: They'll help you fill in the gaps on days you don't meet all your nutrient needs, and are a lifesaver when it comes to those few nutrients needed in levels above and beyond what even a healthful diet can provide (such as calcium, vitamin D, or, for some, vitamin B_{12}). Your need for certain nutrients also changes as you age, and your requirements for some cannot always be met by diet alone.

Someday, your doctor or nutritionist will be able to tailor a supplement to your individual needs based on your genes. But until the science of nutrigenomics (also called nutritional genomics) yields more definitive clues, there are some general recommendations that should be followed. I recommend certain supplements in moderate doses, not exceeding the levels suggested by the Institute of Medicine (IOM), the organization responsible for creating the recommended dietary allowances (RDAs). In most cases, the research does not support a need for higher levels of any one vitamin or mineral, and high doses of some can even be harmful. For instance, you can quickly reach toxic levels of vitamin A (retinol) and certain trace minerals like zinc with indiscriminate use of high-dose or megadose dietary supplements.

You should strive to get all of your nutrients first and foremost from a healthful diet. Supplements should never be used as a substitute for healthy eating. However, a multi can often provide some insurance, especially at certain stages in your life. Some nutrients also require special consideration. I'll discuss them here, too.

Multivitamin and Mineral Supplement

While a multivitamin and mineral supplement may help seal up most of the cracks in your diet, it's not complete in the sense that it doesn't cover you on phytonutrients, nor does it provide fiber or essential omega-3 fats — those you best get from food. It's especially important to take a multivitamin and mineral supplement if you're eating fewer than 1,500 calories a day, you're a vegan or vegetarian, you're highly athletic, or you have had a gastric bypass.

Anti-Aging Hormone Supplementation

One of the natural consequences of aging is a decline in the production of certain hormones, resulting in everything from thinning hair to muscle loss to lack of libido. It stands to reason, then, that adding back hormones in the form of medication or dietary supplements may halt the hormonal effects of aging. But unfortunately, it's not that simple. "There can be side effects that outweigh the benefits," says John J. Merendino, Jr., MD, an assistant clinical professor at the George Washington University School of Medicine. Here's the rundown on the hormone supplements most commonly used in anti-aging treatments.

Human Growth Hormone (hGH)

hGH is made by the pituitary gland at the base of the brain and is essential for normal growth and development, especially during childhood and adolescence. With age, production declines, prompting such effects as loss of muscle mass and an increase in body fat. In studies looking at hGH supplementation, people getting growth hormone have had more muscle mass, less body fat, and an increase in the capacity for aerobic exercise. "But they've also had an increase in certain problems, including arthritis and diabetes," says Dr. Merendino. hGH treatment may help people with a medically related deficiency, but is widely thought to be too risky for normal, aging adults—though there are vocal proponents despite the fact that giving hGH to anyone who is not diagnosed as having a deficiency is not approved by the Food and Drug Administration (FDA). Increased exercise and an improved diet also result in higher hGH levels in healthy adults—without any negative side effects.

Testosterone

Waning testosterone levels in men (and in women) result in a somewhat reduced interest in sex, less muscle mass, and less stamina. So far research looking at supplemental testosterone for normal aging hasn't been too promising. "Most trials have yielded generally disappointing results, with some increase in muscle mass but no clear benefit in terms of bone density, sexual function, or sense of well-being," reports Dr. Merendino. "And there are risks, including a worsening of sleep apnea, prostate enlargement, and possibly excessive red blood cell production, which can lead to stroke."

Hormone Replacement Therapy (HRT)

Whereas testosterone levels decline slowly in healthy men, women undergo a fairly abrupt and significant decline in their sexual hormones — estrogen, progesterone, and, yes, testosterone — at menopause. The estrogenic effects of over-the-counter supplements such as those derived from soy are relatively weak, but what about HRT? Is it safe? Hormone replacement therapy definitely has anti-aging benefits, such as an improvement in bone density and a decrease in hot flashes and the dryness of the vaginal walls that typically occurs with menopause. But there are also fairly clear risks, such as an overall increase in breast cancer and, possibly, heart disease among women on HRT. Weighing the risks and benefits is something best done in conversation with your doctor.

DHEA

The one hormone widely used for its reputed anti-aging effects that can be obtained legally without a prescription in the United States (it's a dietary supplement and therefore doesn't need FDA approval) is DHEA, dihydroepiandrosterone. DHEA is a hormone made by the adrenal glands, and its levels in the bloodstream fall with age in both men and women. By age eighty, most people have about 75 percent less DHEA than they did at age twenty-five. DHEA has testosterone-like effects, and some women who take it get excessive facial or body hair. It also has estrogenic effects, and some men who take it get breast enlargement. It may also interact with hormone receptors in the brain that are important for mood regulation, and many proponents believe that DHEA has antidepressant properties. Yet despite its reputation, data from carefully done studies does not support the idea that DHEA turns back the clock, and studies have also shown that quality control in the production of many commercial DHEA preparations is quite poor. The upshot: pass on DHEA supplements unless your doctor prescribes them.

Research showing the connection between longevity and multis isn't definitive, but it's suggestive. For instance, a Washington State University survey of about 78,000 middle-aged people found that those who took a multi for ten years had a 16 percent lower risk of developing heart disease. However, it's tough to get a read on whether or not multis help stave off age-related diseases or slow the aging process because people who take multis tend to have healthier diets as well. Is it the multi or the diet? Probably a combination of both. When you shop for a multivitamin and mineral supplement, opt for one in which the daily values (DV) of each nutrient are around 100 percent except for those noted below, as well as calcium and magnesium. (The reason multis don't offer more calcium is that the pill would simply be too big to swallow.) Instead of listing all of the recommended levels for each age and gender group on dietary supplement labels, manufacturers use the term DV.

YOUR SUPPLEMENT STRATEGY: Consider taking a standard multivitamin and mineral tablet daily. Here are some tips for finding the right one:

- Look for multivitamins that are formulated at around 100 percent DV for most of the nutrients listed. Some nutrients may be listed at higher than 100 percent — B_1, B_2, and B_{12} are a few examples — but that is okay since they are not toxic at these levels.

- Make sure they have at least 100 percent DV for vitamin D, and for women under 50 years old, 100 percent DV for folic acid.

- Avoid multis with more than 100 percent DV for vitamin A, zinc, and, if you're a woman over 50 or a man of any age, iron.

- Don't be lured by added herbs. There is no evidence that multis with added herbs provide any additional benefits, and they're often a waste of money. Most herbs don't provide any appreciable nutrients, and are present in low quantities or quantities below what might be considered beneficial. Some might also interfere with the absorption of certain nutrients.

- For men, look for a formula with no more than 8 mg iron. For women under 50, look for a formula with at least 18 mg iron. After menopause, a woman's need for iron drops back down to 8 mg, the same amount recommended for men. (This is the primary difference between multi formulas for men versus women, and younger versus older adults.)

Vitamin D

The vitamin D deficiency in this country had been called a "silent epidemic." About 77 percent of Americans have low levels of vitamin D in their blood, according to a government survey. That's worrisome considering how critical D is for building and maintaining bone; helping to prevent cancer, heart disease, and diabetes; and improving immune function. You don't want to be low in D: This is one nutrient with a clear case for supplementation.

Vitamin D is formed when sunlight hits the skin, but if you're not out in the sun much, or use sunscreen or clothing to thwart UV rays (as you should—see page 149), it's easy to fall short. This is especially true if you have dark skin. Melanin protects the skin from the sun, but it also inhibits the skin's ability to synthesize vitamin D. (Light skin, on the other hand, synthesizes D with little exposure, which makes sense on an evolutionary level since lighter-skinned people traditionally lived in the north where light was scarcer.) People who are obese are particularly susceptible to low levels of D, as are older adults who often don't convert sunlight into D efficiently. Because the sun is weaker in winter, it's also possible to have a deficiency during the colder months, especially if you live in northern latitudes (above Denver, St. Louis, San Francisco, or Washington, D.C.)

And you're not going to find much vitamin D occurring naturally in foods. It's in a few types of fish and mushrooms that have been exposed to light (as mentioned earlier, mushrooms purposely grown to be high in vitamin D have begun hitting the market), but otherwise, the D in your diet has to come from fortified milk, or dairy products made with fortified milk (don't assume there is vitamin D in all yogurts and cheeses), some cereals, and spreads made without partially hydrogenated fats (like Bestlife buttery spread and spray).

Studies show that fortified foods do a good job of helping many people meet recommended levels for vitamin D, though scientists are now trying to determine if supplementing with D can give you a disease-prevention edge. One Canadian study of about 6,500 women found that those supplementing with more than 400 IU of vitamin D daily cut their risk of developing breast cancer by 25 percent. Other studies have shown that vitamin D supplementation may help lower the risk of colon cancer, prostate cancer, and even death from any cause. Supplementing with both D and calcium — but not D alone — appears to reduce the risk of bone fractures.

YOUR SUPPLEMENT STRATEGY: Get a blood test to determine your vitamin D level. If you're deficient or have a low level, follow your doctor's recommendation — that might be a high dose (prescription level) of D for a few months to get blood levels back up. Once you're back to a normal level, or if you are already at normal levels, make sure you get a minimum of 600 IU from all sources (supplements and fortified foods, and the few foods containing D) if you're an adult age seventy or younger; 800 IU if you're seventy-one or older. This is consistent with the current IOM recommendation; however, some researchers think it may not be high enough. (Look for reports on vitamin D news as well as updates on all facets of anti-aging nutrition on www.20YearsYounger.com.)

Your multi should give you at least 600 IU (800 IU if you're over age seventy). Try to get much of your D from foods first, and the rest through a vitamin D supplement. If you choose a supplement, look to see that it contains vitamin D_3, which is used more efficiently by the body than D_2.

Calcium

Besides its critical role in building and maintaining bone — especially important as you age and bone turnover slows down — calcium also helps regulate muscle contractions (including contraction of the heart) and blood pressure. Some evidence suggests that calcium protects against colon cancer, too. Calcium works in tandem with vitamin D to assist certain functions in the body, and you need to consume them together in order to absorb the calcium. So, take your calcium supplement at the same time as your multi, or, if you need extra D, take a combined calcium/D supplement.

Given that adults need a lot of calcium — 1,000 mg calcium up to age fifty, then 1,200 mg for women over age fifty and men over age seventy — and most Americans aren't meeting this requirement, taking a supplement is a good idea for many people. You can also meet the requirement with a combination of supplementation and food. The 20 Years Younger meal plan in Part II manages to pack 1,000 mg of calcium into most day's menus, so getting adequate calcium through food is doable. Still, it's not all that easy, especially when you're keeping a lid on calories.

Although bone density peaks in young adulthood it's important to get adequate amounts of calcium and vitamin D throughout your life to keep your bones healthy. In five separate studies in which elderly people took 700 to 800 IU of vitamin D and about 1,000 mg of calcium per day, hip fractures fell by about 24 percent.

YOUR SUPPLEMENT STRATEGY: If you're age fifty or younger, you need 1,000 mg calcium daily. You should meet your needs with food first, then add a calcium supplement. To get 1,000 mg calcium through food, try this mix:

- Consume two cups of nonfat or 1% milk, calcium-fortified soy milk, and/or 1–1½ cups nonfat or low-fat plain yogurt daily (that supplies 600 to 700 mg calcium).
- Eat a wide variety of nutritious foods, a la our meal plan, which contributes another 300 mg calcium.

If you aren't making the entire 1,000 mg through food, I recommend a calcium carbonate supplement (check the label — it will tell you the source of the product's calcium) taken with vitamin D or a combined calcium/D tablet. Take no more than 500 mg of calcium at one time. A good strategy: take one tablet in the a.m. and the other in the p.m.

If you're a woman age fifty-one or older or a man over the age of seventy and getting calcium through food as outlined above, you'll need to add another cup of milk, calcium-fortified soy milk and/or plain yogurt or take a

300-to-500-mg calcium supplement. Also, after age fifty it's a good idea to switch from using a calcium carbonate–based supplement to one made from calcium citrate. As you age, the level of acid in your stomach drops, and in that environment calcium citrate is better absorbed.

Vitamin B$_{12}$

B$_{12}$ and another B vitamin, folate (also called folic acid), are essential for properly functioning DNA and for the creation of certain proteins. Anything that influences DNA influences aging, so getting enough of this vitamin is critical, particularly because a severe deficiency can cause permanent neurological damage to your limbs and brain, and even dementia. Vegans and vegetarians are at risk because B$_{12}$ is found only in animal foods, though you can find it in certain fortified breakfast cereals and soy milks. Consider a supplement if you don't eat meat or eggs. The risk of a B$_{12}$ deficiency goes up in all people after the age of fifty. About 10 to 30 percent of people over the age of fifty have atrophic gastritis, low stomach acid secretion, and stomach acid is required to properly absorb B$_{12}$.

In gauging your B$_{12}$ intake, it's also important to consider how much folic acid you're getting in your diet (the recommended amount is 400 mcg for men and nonpregnant women). Folic acid can affect the blood in a way that makes it difficult for a doctor to tell if you have a B$_{12}$ deficiency. If you're supplementing with folic acid (many women hoping to get pregnant do), you need to supplement with B$_{12}$ as well, no matter what your age. If you take a multi, then you're covered—a good multi like the type we recommend on page 126 will cover you for both. Be aware that if you're eating a lot of foods that are fortified with folic acid, you may be tipping the balance and getting a lot more folic acid than B$_{12}$. It's possible that you may not even be aware that you're eating folic acid–enriched foods. In 1996, in an effort to make sure pregnant women got enough folic acid (it prevents neural tube birth defects), the FDA published regulations requiring the addition of folic acid to enriched breads, cereals, flours, cornmeals, pastas, rice, and other grain products. Thus, many carbohydrates that you may eat on a regular basis contain added folic

Countering Macular Degeneration with Supplements

Macular degeneration, the leading cause of blindness in the United States, begins with blurring in the center of your field of vision and can progress to total blindness. At age sixty, you've got a 2 percent risk of getting it; after age seventy-five your risk jumps to 30 percent. It's unknown whether dietary supplements can help prevent macular degeneration from developing—to tell for sure, people would have to supplement from childhood throughout life, which is very costly. But there's research suggesting that people who take multivitamin/mineral tablets for at least ten years have a lower risk of developing the disease. The longer the multi is taken, the better the protection.

It's clear that once you get macular degeneration, supplements can slow its progression. In AREDS (Age-Related Eye Disease Study) people with the intermediate stage of macular degeneration given 500 mg of vitamin C, 400 IU vitamin E, 15 mg beta-carotene, 80 mg zinc, and 2 mg copper were 25 percent less likely to progress to advanced macular degeneration in a five-year period. The study is being continued without beta-carotene because of the link between beta-carotene and increased cancer risk (see page 134).

Even though the AREDS study couldn't discern whether taking the supplements helps at early stages of macular degeneration, talk to your doctor to see if it's appropriate for you to take specially formulated AREDS supplements. They're available from companies such as Icap and Bausch and Lomb (Ocuvite).

acid. However, whole grain versions usually aren't fortified—another reason to switch to whole grains.

YOUR SUPPLEMENT STRATEGY: The RDA for B_{12} for all adults is 2.4 mcg daily. Most standard multis provide more—about 6 mcg—and it's the amount you should be getting if you're age fifty or younger to help counter all the folic acid that's been added to foods. If you're over age fifty, you might also consider taking a vitamin B_{12} supplement with at least 50 mcg. It sounds high, but it's a safe dose, and helps ensure that you're getting enough if you've been diagnosed with atrophic gastritis. Either an oral or a sublingual (under the tongue) B_{12} supplement will do the trick.

Supplement Safety

While certain types of supplements may be helpful, there are some circumstances when supplements can actually be harmful. Here's what you should know before you shop.

If you're prone to kidney stones, be careful with calcium. Ask your doctor before taking calcium and vitamin D supplements. Most kidney stones are a mix of calcium and oxalates—compounds found in a variety of plants such as tea and whole grains. For people prone to kidney stones, taking in too much calcium can trigger stone formation. Yet even if you have a tendency to develop kidney stones, you still need to get adequate calcium. Some studies show that supplementing with calcium may actually protect against forming stones but only when the supplements are taken *with* a meal. This strategy reduces the likelihood of kidney stone formation because you absorb more calcium when you consume it with food. Take them outside of a meal and more winds up in the kidneys, where there's a greater likelihood of the calcium binding with oxalates and forming stones.

In addition to taking calcium supplements with a meal, spread out your dose through the day, taking no more than 500 mg calcium at a time as noted earlier; that should prevent any problems. We also know that consuming plenty of fluids is one of the best ways to reduce your risk of kidney stones. Reducing your sodium intake might also be helpful because sodium in high amounts (the amount typically consumed by most Americans) can leech calcium out of your bones and the calcium eventually ends up in your kidneys.

Since vitamin D helps your body absorb calcium, high doses may impair kidney function by causing too much calcium to be absorbed. But it takes a lot of vitamin D—50,000 IU daily—to cause this problem.

If you've been diagnosed with precancerous colon polyps, cap folic acid at 400 mcg per day or less. Some research indicates that supplementation may actually spur polyps to become cancerous. Though folic acid is generally protective against cancer because it helps repair DNA and promotes growth of healthy cells, in excess, that same mechanism might trigger the growth of any cancer cells lurking. The research is still very preliminary, so it's unclear at what point in your life you should avoid excess folic acid, and how much is too much if you have polyps (what we *do* know is that the upper limit for everybody is 1,000 mcg per day).

Because most multis offer 100 percent of the daily value for folic acid, consider taking it every other day if you are also consuming a lot of fortified foods. Missing out on all the other vitamins and minerals a multi provides every other day shouldn't pose a problem for you if you're consuming a healthy diet. The only exception is vitamin D, and for that I recommend taking a separate supplement. Before you decide to switch to taking a multi every other day instead of daily, check labels to find out which foods in your diet are fortified with folic acid, particularly labels of cereals, breads, and energy bars. (See page 130 for more on preventing folic acid overload.)

Even if you haven't any reason to think you've got precancerous polyps in the colon, sticking to no more than 400 mcg of folic acid daily is probably wise, especially if you are over age fifty. As noted earlier, another reason to avoid high doses at that age is that too much folic acid can cover up a vitamin B_{12} deficiency, to which people over age fifty are prone. Meanwhile, continue to eat foods *naturally* high in folate such as oranges and spinach — all the evidence points to naturally occurring folate as being protective. If you are under age fifty and plan to become pregnant, or if you are currently pregnant, you need to supplement with at least 400 mcg of folic acid daily. This is essential for helping to prevent a neural tube defect in your child and trumps concerns about colon cancer.

Avoid supplementing with beta-carotene beyond levels in a standard multi. Beta-carotene is an antioxidant plant pigment that gives plant foods such as carrots and cantaloupe their orange color and is also found in dark green vegetables. Your body converts beta-carotene, alpha-carotene, and a few other carotenoids to vitamin A as needed. Numerous studies show that people with high levels of beta-carotene in their diet and in their blood have a lower risk of cancer, so researchers figured that supplementing with it might help ward off the disease.

That's when they got a big surprise. In two large studies, beta-carotene supplements were given to smokers and asbestos workers, the people most prone to lung cancer. Instead of offering protection as hoped, the beta-carotene supplementation increased the incidence of lung cancer and death. As for other cancers—such as pancreatic, breast, and prostate—the beta-carotene had no effect.

Fruits and vegetables that contain beta-carotene are also infused with other carotenoids and nutrients that work synergistically with one another to promote health. Removing beta-carotene from the food and delivering it alone in pill form does not have the same effect as consuming it in foods.

The take-home: Getting beta-carotene through food is important. However, while moderate levels of beta-carotene in your multi are safe (3 to 6 mg of beta-carotene daily, the equivalent of 833 IU to 1,667 IU vitamin A is fine) and probably helpful, don't take separate beta-carotene supplements. A typical multi splits up vitamin A between beta-carotene and straight-out vitamin A (retinol). Check the back of the bottle—ideally, the multi should contain no more than 4,000 IU of vitamin A total, with no more than 50 percent beta-carotene.

Avoid supplementing with vitamin E in amounts greater than 200 IU. Vitamin E, like beta-carotene, looked so promising as a safeguard against cancer and heart disease. It's also a powerful antioxidant. Some studies have shown that E from food and supplement sources may improve your chances of staving off heart disease. But in 2005, a review of the research found that in nine out of eleven major studies in which people took 400 IU or more of vitamin E from supplements alone, not only was it *not* protective, but it seemed to actually increase the risk of heart failure, gastrointestinal cancer, and dying from any cause—the more vitamin E, the higher the risk. Other research has confirmed the results and even shown that E supplements may slightly increase the risk of stroke. How to make sense of it all? It may be that the study subjects were taking too much vitamin E. Or too little: In one study, most of the deaths occurred in "noncompliant" people who didn't actually take their vitamin E tablet as they were supposed to.

And there are still studies showing that vitamin E may improve your chances of staving off heart disease. For instance, in the Harvard's Women's Health Trial, which had 20,000 women taking 600 IU of vitamin E or a placebo every other day for ten years, there was a 24 percent drop in deaths from heart disease in women over age sixty-five taking vitamin E as compared to those taking the placebo (for younger women, there was no effect). While it's safe to take as much as 400 IU of vitamin E daily, the evidence suggests that a lower amount, about 200 IU, may be more beneficial. Most multis only have about 30 IU, so a separate supplement might be appropriate (especially if your diet is lacking). Buy the natural form (d-alpha-tocopherol) and take it with a meal; otherwise it may not get absorbed into your system. If you find that it's nearly as expensive to buy 200 IU tablets as 400 IU, then buy the latter and take a pill every other day.

Because supplements are sold over the counter, it's easy to assume that they are all safe and beneficial. Not necessarily so. To sum up, here is what you should keep in mind when you shop.

- Multivitamin and mineral supplements can be helpful, but make sure that you purchase one that is well balanced.

- Never megadose — that is, take double or triple (or more) of the levels recommended by the Institute of Medicine — even if you've read that a vitamin or mineral has no known toxicity.

- If you have any type of health condition, always discuss supplementation with your doctor before stocking up.

- Always bring a list of supplements you are taking with you when you see your doctor. Some supplements can interfere with certain drugs, and your doctor needs to know what you're taking when prescribing medications for you — or even when diagnosing your condition.

CHAPTER 4

Recapturing Your Skin's Youth

By Harold A. Lancer, MD, FAAD

THERE ARE ALL KINDS OF THINGS you can do to make your skin *look* younger — but why bother creating an illusion when, with a good skin care routine, you can make your skin actually *be* younger? I'm talking about a true turning back of the clock. As you restore good health to your skin, all the machinery that's slowed down due to natural aging or damaging environmental effects (such as the sun) will kick back into gear, creating real physiological changes. Your skin will behave like its former, more metabolically upbeat self. As a result, it can be firmer, smoother, more uniform in color, and altogether more radiant.

Whether skin "looks" young or "acts" young might seem like splitting hairs, but there's a significant difference between *the appearance* of young skin and skin that frequently and naturally refreshes itself, regularly churns out the fibers that give it structure and elasticity, and rapidly repairs itself when necessary — all hallmarks of youthful, undamaged skin. Let me put it to you this way: You can slip into a pair of Spanx to disguise a flabby belly, but that doesn't make you fit and slim. Once you slip out of the Spanx, there is that flabby belly, back again. In the same way, you can rub a moisturizer onto your skin and get it looking dewy and even give yourself a bit of a glow. Or apply makeup that deflects light, drawing attention away from the lines and wrinkles on your face. But these are fleeting, superficial solutions. What you really want to do is change what's going on *beneath* the surface of your skin so that you get it working properly again, just like it used to work twenty years ago. A proper skin hygiene program is truly age reversing. And, in most cases, no involved procedures are necessary.

YOUTH AND BEAUTY

Your skin, of course, is the cover of the "book" of who you really are. It gives clues to your inner physical and psychological self. But if we're honest about it, we primarily pursue that youthful appearance because in all cultures, youthfulness is synonymous with beauty and beauty is synonymous with good health, fertility, success, and a good life.

Although beauty is in the eye of the beholder (and never has a greater truth been spoken), I think you'd be hard pressed to find anyone who doesn't admire smooth, glowing skin. It's universally held by every culture, every ethnicity, both genders, and the wealthy and the less fortunate that firm, resilient, even-toned, radiant skin communicates well-being and beauty. Good skin is sexy. *Great skin is sexier!* It's your best calling card, the attribute that's going to make the most indelible impression on everyone you meet.

One way you can recognize well-maintained skin is by its radiant glow. When it's in top form, light skin will have a rosy gleam to it; dark skin will look luminous. This is a sign that the skin is getting adequate blood flow and is readily replenishing and repairing itself. So if you want to look twenty years younger, you need to go for the glow. And the bounce. Universally admired skin also has elasticity. Push gently and it will rebound without a mark. It has a healthy fullness to it, too. How plump is the pillow? Are all the feathers in there and fully fluffed? And what do the pores look like? Small (the more imperceptible, the better), uniform pores are the gold standard in skin, a sign that it's looking and acting young.

I'm not just talking about the skin on your face. Most people think skin care starts at the hairline and stops at the chin, but if you think about it, and especially if you're a woman, your neck and chest area are often just as exposed to the perceptive public. I tell my patients that the neck, chest, and shoulders (as well as the upper part of the back, if you want to be completely thorough) frame the face, and that those areas deserve the exact same tender loving care. Sometimes I'll see a patient who needs to pay more attention to her neck-chest zone than to her face, no doubt the result of having spent years lavishing care from the chin up while ignoring everything beneath it. *All* areas of your body, right down to your fingertips, should reflect the same maintenance and repair. Environmental damage happens all over, so I'm going to be reminding you again and again not to forget the terrain beneath your chin. Get the glow and make sure it extends down below!

SMART, MODERN, DO-IT-YOURSELF SKIN CARE

Despite what you may have heard, there is no one miracle in a bottle, magic-bullet ingredient, dramatic procedure, or highly elaborate regimen that will reverse aging. What it takes instead is a combination of the healthy practices outlined throughout this book — regular exercise, nutritious eating, and good sleep — with a simple, at-home, anti-aging skin care plan. You don't need to spend a lot of money and you don't need to spend a whole day caring for yourself. Simplicity will get you cost-effective, visible results from head to toe.

You'll notice that I said "skin care." This do-it-yourself approach is a new way of thinking about anti-aging as it relates to appearance. It's been a long time since anyone talked about home-based skin care. Instead, people concerned about aging are being urged to make a beeline to the nearest purveyor of line fillers and wrinkle-freezers, or to head for a clinic offering skin resurfacing laser treatments. It's not uncommon for patients to come in for the first time and ask straight away for Botox or a laser procedure that a friend had done, without any thought to their own particular needs. I think that's a big mistake, and I always ask them to at least start with good skin hygiene before advancing to the next step. Though there is a place for doctors' office peels, injectables, and laser treatments, you probably won't need any of them if you have an effective skin care program like the one I'm going to introduce you to. And, while there are famous faces that have obviously "had work done" (and then some!), I think you'd be surprised at how many lovely, glowing faces you see on the screen, in business, and in politics that are attributable to nothing but a proper method of skin care. And this seems to be a growing trend.

What constitutes good skin hygiene? The method I developed for my patients involves three basic steps for your face, neck, and chest—polishing the skin, cleansing it, then nourishing it—and two steps for your body, hands, and feet. The simple steps I recommend work to make the skin biologically more youthful in many ways, including by boosting the circulation in the skin so it receives more oxygen and reparative nutrients, revving up the turnover of skin cells to banish dullness and dryness, and rousing the sleepy collagen- and elastin-making factories to diminish lines and wrinkles.

There are a few reasons why this system is different from others and why it works so well, but foremost is the fact that it targets the stratum corneum, the outermost part of the epidermis, which is the top layer of the skin. Almost every product and procedure you hear about targets the dermis, the layer of the skin that lies below the epidermis. A lot of skin repair does take place in the dermis. However, when you focus solely on that layer, you miss the boat; not much reparative activity can take place if you ignore the stratum corneum. I'll tell you more about the physiology of the skin beginning on page 142, but in brief, the stratum corneum has long been thought of as an inactive, virtually plastic film covering the dynamic parts of the skin. Now we know that many of the signals that generate anatomical change in the skin come from the cells in the stratum corneum. What's more, in order for active ingredients to get into the dermis, they must have a clear path through that top layer.

To that end, the first two steps in the anti-aging skin care method I'll be introducing to you clear away impenetrable debris (a combination of dead skin cells, cosmetics, and dirt) that's accumulated on the surface of the skin, allowing the nourishing components in step three a direct route into the lower layers. When those nourishing ingredients are able to get in and do their work, significant change occurs.

The most important thing about this method is that…it works! But of no small consequence is that it also allows you to fight aging while still maintaining aspects of your appearance that reflect who you are. You still look like *you*. To most of the patients over the age of forty that I see in my office, that's essential. I've never had a patient tell me that she'd like to look eighteen again. What I do commonly hear is "I simply want to look healthy — because I *am* healthy. I just want my skin to reflect that." Many people I talk to have also seen the consequences of being overstretched, overplumped, or over-neutralized and they know that's not what they want. Instead, they want to look refreshed — like a more rested version of themselves — and they want to take an active role in caring for their skin. They see it as part of taking control of their own overall well-being, and they're right: Committing to good skin care goes hand in hand with committing to the other strategies in this book for achieving total body health.

Sticking to the polish-cleanse-nourish method is something anyone can fit into his or her life. And if you like, you can also go further, taking it to the next level by adding other, more specialized (but still simple) steps to deal with specific problems like deep lines, acne, rosacea, or excessive dryness. After you see improvements in your complexion from consistent care, you may even find that you have the desire for greater changes. Dermatologist-provided anti-aging "touch-ups" — chemical peels, laser treatments, and injectables — can be part of a healthy skin care regimen, too, as long as the procedures you have done are appropriate to your particular skin and executed with care. But I would never recommend that you seek any interventions without first trying the three-step method in this book.

What you put on your skin is important. Lotions, creams, exfoliators, toners, serums, and so on, provided you choose good ones, can have a visible impact on your skin. But I don't believe they are as important as the *method* of skin care you use. The right method — that is, the polish-cleanse-nourish method — both stimulates changes in the skin and ensures that the therapeutic compounds you put on it hit their targets. You can have the best skin care products in the world, but if the active ingredients can't get into the deeper layers of the skin, they'll simply sit there on the surface, inert and ineffective. The skin hygiene secret is in the sequencing — puzzle solved!

The method I'm going to tell you about is uncomplicated and requires very little actual time to complete — but you do have to stick to the routine without fail. And you can't depend on polishing, cleansing, and nourishing alone. Staying out of the sun, shedding the tobacco habit, reducing your alcohol intake, eating a more selective diet, developing a regular exercise program, striving for significant and restful sleep, and, finally, managing stress, are all important as well. So is drinking at least six glasses of water a day, and by water I don't mean a beverage that contains water like coffee or iced tea. (I can always tell which of my patients have fallen off the "lifestyle wagon" by the quality of their skin.) When you have all these proactive and precautionary measures in place, you're going to see a real turnaround in the health of your skin. Let's talk about why.

YOUR SKIN, UNCOVERED

I like to call skin your "best accessory" because, while a stunning ring or a striking scarf or a great watch attracts attention, nothing catches the eye quite like beautiful skin. But the truth is, as the body's largest organ and with miles and miles of capillaries and nerves, millions of oil and sweat glands, and countless hair follicles and cells all communicating with one another, skin is more like an entire outfit. It's all-encompassing, a community unto itself.

Understanding a little bit about the anatomy of skin can help you better grasp the changes you've seen as you've gotten older, as well as give you a clearer picture of how certain techniques, products, and procedures work to change how it functions. As you might guess, the skin is a very complex organ, and it's not necessary to know how every sweat gland and blood vessel works. So let's just go over the parts of the skin's makeup that are both instrumental in aging and particularly responsive to anti-aging measures.

If you were to look under a microscope at a tiny swath of skin, you'd see layer upon layer upon layer. The stratum corneum alone, which is the utmost top of the skin, has more than twenty layers. It's easiest, though, to think of

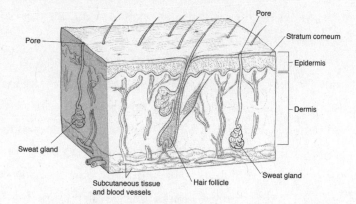

the skin as divided into three parts: the epidermis with its top "sheet," the stratum corneum; the dermis; and the subcutaneous tissue.

Stratum Corneum

Glance down at your hand. What you're looking at is the stratum corneum, a brick-and-mortar construction of flat, tightly packed cells called keratino-cytes (the bricks) enveloped in lipids (the mortar). The stratum corneum is thicker on the areas of the body that need greater protection, such as the soles of the feet and palms of the hands.

In some ways this topmost layer (or layers, really) functions a little like a raincoat, keeping excessive moisture and harmful microbes and environ-mental toxins out. However it also has the very important task of keeping adequate moisture *in* the skin. It does this with the help of a biological stew of amino acids and other elements, including one called natural moisturiz-ing factor (NMF). NMF absorbs water from the atmosphere, keeping the stra-tum corneum soft and preventing it from developing cracks.

Although they still serve an important purpose, by the time keratino-cytes reach the surface of the skin, they are actually dead cells. They're cre-ated in the layers beneath the stratum corneum, then work their way to the top, aging and dying along the way. This process — called cell turnover — can take anywhere from twenty-six to forty-two days. Like shells washing up on the shore of a beach, the dead cells arrive at the very top layer of the stratum corneum, where they're routinely sloughed off. It's this sloughing-off process that helps the skin stay radiant.

When cell turnover slows down, which it does naturally with age and also as a result of injury such as sun damage or a lack of moisture in the skin, the old cells stick together and accumulate on the surface. That's why older or injured skin often looks lackluster and the reason it becomes more impenetrable, making it harder for therapeutic skin care products to do their job.

The good news is that though the stratum corneum is made up of primarily "dead" cells, it is far from a lifeless entity. When properly stimulated and cleared of the very top cells, it sends various signals down to the layers below, among them orders for increased production of new cells. When that occurs, cell renewal speeds up again and the skin regains its glow.

Epidermis

One of the main activities going on in the epidermis is the production of compounds that keep the skin hydrated. The epidermis is where NMF and fats such as cholesterol, triglycerides, and ceramides are produced, then used to create the "mortar" in the stratum corneum.

The epidermis is also a melanin-making factory. Melanin, otherwise known as pigment, is made by cells called melanocytes. It not only colors the skin and hair, but it helps protect against damage from ultraviolet (UV) rays. The more melanin you have (and thus the darker in appearance your skin and hair), the more protection against UV rays your skin will provide. So skin actually has its own sunscreen—but not nearly enough, especially white skin. Black skin has been shown to have a sun protection factor (SPF) of 13.4, whereas light Caucasian skin has only an SPF of 3.4. Yet no matter where you fall on that spectrum, you don't want to depend solely on your natural SPF. Everyone should wear sunscreen, and I'll talk about it at length beginning on page 163. Also bear in mind that, except in small areas where it forms age spots, the amount of melanin produced in the epidermis decreases with age, which can give the skin a pallor. Tanning, though, isn't the answer to restoring vibrancy to your complexion—it actually has the opposite effect.

Dermis

The dermis is home to the primary scaffolding of the skin: collagen, proteins that give the skin shape and durability; and elastin, proteins that give it resilience. Primary production of these structural protein fibers grinds to a halt at about age twenty-five, the reason skin begins to lose its bounce and fullness and starts forming lines and wrinkles. With age and environmental offenders such as the sun, collagen and elastin break down, causing an even greater loss of the healthy plumpness that makes skin look smooth and unlined. It shouldn't be surprising, then, that a lot of anti-aging skin care is aimed at "waking up" fibroblasts, the cells that create collagen and elastin.

Fibroblasts in the dermis also produce compounds called glycosaminoglycans (GAGs). GAGs are gel-like and form the "soup" in which the collagen and elastin reside. As the production of GAGs slows with age, the cushioning in the skin that they form flattens out and causes the skin to wrinkle and depreciate. Since GAGs — and in particular one called hyaluronic acid — also help the skin hold on to water, their loss can make the skin dry and flaky.

Woven into the dermis are sweat glands, nerve endings, and blood vessels that bring nutrients to the skin and remove wastes. Hair follicles also originate in the dermis and are connected to the sebaceous glands, which create the oily substance sebum. Sebum helps keep the skin soft and impervious to water, and it's also one of the culprits behind acne. When sebum is overproduced, it clogs the hair follicles and pores (through which it's secreted) and mixes with bacteria, causing an angry inflammatory response.

Subcutaneous Fat

Aside from providing insulation and cushioning, the subcutaneous fat layer gives the skin volume and shape. You may want to lose fat in other areas of your body, but not here. Unfortunately, the subcutaneous layer does shift and diminish as the years go by, causing certain areas of the face and other parts of the body to sag. Folds near the nose (called nasolabial folds), jowls, and wrinkles are all related to the movement and loss of subcutaneous fat.

SKIN DIFFERENCES AMONG INDIVIDUALS

The specific makeup of your skin will reflect your ancestral heritage as well as your gender and lifestyle. Black skin, for instance, tends to have a thicker stratum corneum and dermis, a denser fabric of collagen and elastin fibers, and more tightly packed pores, oil glands, and sweat glands than white skin. For all these reasons—and because greater melanin content makes people of color less susceptible to the ravages of UV rays—dark skin shows less conventional signs of aging. However, dark skin has a much more reactive biology than light skin, leading to different problems with skin repair. For this reason, dark skin often scars rapidly and dramatically.

Brown skin, such as that of people of Asian, Mediterranean, Middle Eastern, Latin American, and American Indian heritage as well as combined ethnicities, typically has the best of both worlds. It shares a similar structure with black skin, which makes it visually age more slowly, and, like white skin, it's generally much less likely to scar. Brown skin also responds somewhat more predictably to lasers and other procedures than black skin.

There are some slight differences between male and female skin, too. Men usually have thicker skin, more collagen and elastin tissue, and more sweat and oil glands than women. However, men also tend to get more exposure to the elements, so any advantage they have in skin construction is often canceled out by environmental factors. It's sometimes thought that men don't show their age as obviously as women, but I'm inclined to believe that's more perception than reality. Some of the most successful movie actors have craggy, timeworn faces; an actress who wore her age as noticeably would be lucky to get a walk-on part. I believe that's simply because we're more accepting of facial aging in men than in women—not because men age better.

HOW THE SKIN AGES

True or false: Lines, wrinkles, and all the other hallmarks of aging skin are just a sign that nature is taking its course. The answer is true *and* false (I admit, it

---

Skin Care Mistake #1

Going to Sleep with Makeup On

You've already had your makeup on all day, what harm could a few more hours do? As it turns out, a lot. All cosmetic products that provide color and illusion leave a toxic chemical film on the skin's surface that can cause irritation, inflammation, dehydration, and clogged pores. No matter how tired you are at night, take the time to meticulously wash your face, neck, and chest.

---

was a bit of a trick question). Here's the part that's true. Some of the aspects of aging are unavoidable; you might say they're part of the human condition. And genetics certainly plays a role, so if your parents' skin aged well, yours may age nicely, too (and, of course, if their skin aged badly there's an increased likelihood that yours won't fare so well either). So, yes, in some sense, lines, wrinkles, sagging, dryness, dullness, spider veins—all that is just nature doing what nature does. That's called intrinsic ("from inside") aging.

However, in most people, the degree to which those signs of aging I just mentioned are apparent is determined by environmental factors—things such as sun exposure, smoking, diet, air pollution, and other things that you frequently have some control over. That's called extrinsic ("from outside") aging, and it can even override genetics to some degree. Your skin may behave like your mother's in almost all respects, but if she's a smoker and you've never indulged, she may end up far more wrinkled than you. Conversely, if she avoided the sun all her life and you sunbathed in the yard with a reflector every summer of your teens and twenties, you're not likely to have as smooth a visage as your mom.

Generally, intrinsic and extrinsic aging combine to give you the face you see in the mirror. I have a ninety-five-year-old patient who illustrates the point beautifully. This woman is some kind of English royalty and she has been pampered since birth. She has outlived four, maybe five husbands and is always asking me to set her up on dates, though she won't date anyone over sixty-five. But here's the thing: She could be sixty-five herself. She's never really been in the sun and her skin is smooth, pink, and baby fresh.

There is not a single brown spot on her face. She has never had surgery, laser resurfacing, or chemical peeling, although she does religiously follow the skin care recommendations I've given her. There is one area in which my patient does show signs that she's a "woman of a certain age": volume — everything that contributes to the skin looking full and taut like a well-filled balloon. The plumpness of her skin has depreciated, creating some sagging and folds. Given her age, I'd say that my patient still has a genetic predisposition to slow volume loss, but she, like everyone, couldn't avoid it altogether. Even so, her meticulous care of her skin all these years has paid off.

Let's take a closer look at how some intrinsic and extrinsic factors age the skin.

Genetics and Volume Loss

Genetics holds a lot of sway over how well you fare in the natural aging process. Some people's cell turnover doesn't slow down as quickly as others', and their skin is simply better equipped to weather insults such as sun and pollution than people from a less fortunate gene pool. Their telomeres, the end pieces of chromosomes that help keep cells healthy, are long, and their bodies are inherently good at repairing cell DNA. And, as I discussed on page 146, they may have a slower-aging racial heritage in their favor.

I see the biggest influence of genetics on my patients in the amount of volume they lose from their faces as they grow older. I believe that about 80 percent of the depreciation of soft tissue, particularly in the face, is intrinsic. Even if you care for your skin as well as my ninety-five-year-old patient, there is not much you can do with skin care products alone to stop volume loss from happening. (You can, though, fill the "pillow" back up with injectables.)

Depreciation of collagen and elastin as well as the gel-like GAGs they swim in contributes to volume loss, but the real culprit is the shifting and decline of fat in the subcutaneous layer. In other words, it's not the pillowcase; it's the feathers inside. Some bone loss and changes in muscle can occur, too, further collapsing the structure beneath the epidermis.

Together with gravity and years and years of facial expressions, these factors alter your features and even the shape of your face. A youthful face is an inverted pyramid, with peaked cheeks and the chin as the pinnacle. As the cheeks start melting downward—the air is let out of the balloon—an older face tends to look more like a regular pyramid. The nose can also look bigger with volume loss (partly because the cheeks are smaller), and even the position of the eyebrows can shift.

More marks of the natural aging process:

- thinner, more fragile skin
- drier, mottled skin
- wrinkles, furrows
- fine lines
- lack of bounce
- increased pore size
- lack of uniformity of color
- loss of luminescence

Sun, the #1 Ager

Think, for a minute, of a few classic types. On the one hand, you've got the Irish rose, someone who, living in northern climes, has had little sun exposure. On the other hand, you have the rugged cow wrangler, the person who has spent virtually a lifetime outdoors in the heat. One is blessed with near flawless skin; the other's face is as tough and wrinkled as an old leather jacket. Need I say anything more? Well, actually, I do need to say more, because many people still don't get (or maybe don't care) how insidious the sun really is.

Your skin's deepening in color when exposed to the sun is a sign that UV rays are not welcome. A tan occurs when the epidermis and dermis produce more melanin as a way of protecting the skin against UV damage. (Sunburn is a sign that UV damage has already occurred—skin turns red when living cells in the epidermis and dermis become damaged.) But melanin can only protect you so much. UVB rays, those responsible for sunburn and tanning, penetrate deeply into the skin, but UVA rays go further, and once they get there, they create free radicals, rogue forms of oxygen that degrade collagen and elastin and make it difficult for the skin to rebuild them. Free radicals caused by sun exposure also create something known as cross-linking: chemical bridges between protein molecules in the skin. This makes the skin harder and less elastic (think again of that leathery cowboy) and contributes to the development of wrinkles.

Something else you should know about UVA rays is that they're sneaky — they stream right through glass. Along with UVBs, they're the primary cause of age spots, raised clumps of pigment or other skin cells often found on the hands but which can crop up anywhere on the body. As further insult, UV rays thin the blood vessel walls so that they bleed and show through the skin. The blood vessels also dilate when collagen breaks down, causing red blotchiness to appear, too.

The darker your skin, the more protection your own melanin is going to afford you. However, even if you have very dark skin, UV light and heat still create damaging free radicals. And *all* types of skin are susceptible to sun-induced skin cancer, which I'll talk more about on page 164.

More marks of sun damage:

- skin discoloration
- uneven texture

Smoking and Oxygen Flow

Did you know that the skin of people who smoke takes longer to heal? Nicotine narrows the blood vessels in the skin, depriving it of the oxygen and nutrients it needs to repair itself. But the damage doesn't stop there. Like sunshine, cigarette smoke degrades collagen and elastin and creates free radicals that harm skin cell DNA (air pollution can have this effect, too). Plus, every time smokers drag on a cigarette, they pucker up, an action that, over time, deepens the vertical lines above the lips.

You can really see the difference between smokers and nonsmokers, and researchers at Case Western Reserve University in Cleveland have done a good job of documenting that difference in several studies on twins. In one particularly striking case study, they looked at fifty-two-year-old identical twins, who had always lived in the same town, had about the same amount of sun exposure, and even had the same job. The difference between them is that one was about a pack-a-day smoker while the other never smoked. When you look at pictures of the two women, that difference is clear: On a photo damage (sun damage) scale of 1 to 5, the smoker was a 5 while the non-smoking twin received a grade of 2. In photographs of the two women, the smoking twin has much deeper lines on her cheeks and above the lips — she looks at least ten years older than her sister.

More marks of damage from smoking:

- an unhealthy pallor

- wrinkling all over the body

- dry skin

Acne, Rosacea, and Stress

Acne? Probably about 20 percent of the people I see in my office never had adolescent or teen acne, yet now here they are in middle age as pimply as a sophomore on a prom date, crying, "It's not fair. I get acne and wrinkles at the same time!" They're right. It isn't fair, but it can happen, and the culprit is the same one that bedevils kids: hormones. As menopause approaches, estrogen levels fluctuate, tipping the estrogen-testosterone balance in favor of testosterone. Testosterone pumps up the skin's sebum-making machinery, causing an overproduction of oil that can ultimately clog the hair follicles and pores and trigger breakouts. Estrogen can help modulate the inflammation caused by acne, but when your estrogen levels dip as they do in menopause, you have less natural protection from breakouts.

Some people are also surprised to find that they develop rosacea as they

Skin Care Mistake #2

Locking Yourself in to One Skin Type

Patients always ask me, "What's my skin type?" I can tell them what their skin type is at that moment, in that location, during those particular weather conditions, but I can't tell them what their skin type will be when they fly to Miami the next day or even what their skin type will be later that afternoon. What I'm getting at is that skin type changes from day to day, hour to hour. In the morning you might be dry and flaky, by noon greasy with larger-looking pores. The weather outside, indoor heat and air conditioning, dietary changes, a bout of exercise, the menstrual cycle—all these things can change your skin "type." (One exception is sensitive skin. If products and inclement weather conditions easily irritate your complexion, see page 161.)

I know this can make skin care a little complicated, but it's also the reality. Still, if you keep your routine simple and stay open to amending it when necessary, you should be able to cope. If you buy products for one skin type, choose "combination skin" or the kind that lines up with your usual skin type, then be prepared to treat problems as they happen. If, for instance, your normally dry skin turns oily, a toner can be useful. If you become ruddy, a redness relief product will fit the bill. If your skin becomes dry, you may need a fortified moisturizer. Get to know how your skin behaves at different times and in different locations so that you can tailor your program accordingly.

get older. Rosacea is a chronic condition characterized by redness and inflammation typically caused by swollen blood vessels (primarily on the face, although sometimes in other places, too). In some people, the skin becomes dry and flaky, in others, oily and pimply. Rosacea usually develops between the ages of thirty and fifty and is more common in women and fair-skinned people. It's thought to be passed along in families, and it's far from rare—about 14 million Americans suffer from rosacea. Early signs of rosacea can include flushing when you drink alcohol and facial swelling, small visible bumps on the face and watery or irritated eyes. It's important to see your dermatologist if you suspect you have rosacea, because it's tricky to treat. It makes the skin extremely sensitive and it can be debilitating. One study found that 41 percent of people with rosacea said the condition caused them to avoid going out in public.

Acne and rosacea have a few things in common, and one of them is that stress almost always makes it worse. As part of the response to stress, the adrenal glands, ovaries, and skin produce more testosterone, stimulating the sebaceous glands, which can lead to breakouts. The skin may then become inflamed and heal slowly—two other conditions linked to the stress response. Stress can also impair the skin's barrier function, making it easier for irritants to get in and moisture to get out. That's one reason that stress also makes rosacea worse. In a survey of seven hundred rosacea-sufferers by the National Rosacea Society, 91 percent reported that their condition flares up when they're stressed.

Another way stress may play a role in acne is by encouraging poor eating habits. Many people toss all dietary caution to the wind when they're under pressure, and although there aren't specific foods (chocolate included) that cause acne, some evidence suggests that a high glycemic and low protein diet can worsen existing breakouts. And diet does potentially have a significant influence on the complexion, so healthy eating is imperative for healthy skin. (For more on how diet affects the skin, check my website www .lancerskincare.com.)

Given the connection of stress to acne and rosacea, relaxation techniques such as meditation and yoga, as well as going on vacations—anything that helps ease the pressure of your daily life—can go a long way toward keeping your skin healthy. Lower your stress level and you'll lower the wear and tear on your complexion, too.

AS EASY AS ONE, TWO, THREE: POLISH, CLEANSE, NOURISH

Just about every dermatologist has a story about a patient who, in response to the request "Show me what you're using on your skin," drags in a suitcase full of skin care products. There is absolutely no need to spend extreme amounts of time or money on caring for your skin. If you've got three good products—a polisher (exfoliant), a cleanser, and a nourisher (a topical cream, lotion, serum, oil, or mist with botanical or synthetic anti-aging ingredients such as antioxidants, amino acids, and vitamins)—plus a sunscreen, and take the time to perform three quick steps, once in the morning and once before you go to bed at night, you will be on the path to younger acting and younger looking skin.

Skin care is relatively uncomplicated. Choosing products, unfortunately, isn't quite as simple. The sheer number of anti-aging products on drugstore shelves is staggering. Add to that products sold in department stores, spas, and doctors' offices and the choices become truly mind-boggling. Despite the vast array of options, I often had trouble finding exactly what I was looking for in many skin care products. They either didn't deliver on their promises, didn't work for all of my patients, or required an elaborate regimen. What was missing was combined simplicity and efficacy, so I set out to fill the gap by creating my own line of products, LANCER$_x$ (lancerskincare.com). The products were years in the making, and incorporate some ideas of my own, such as pairing reparative ingredients with oxygenating ingredients that increase their effectiveness. I put a lot of time and effort into developing the products, and I didn't skimp on anything: The ingredients are of the highest quality, used in therapeutic amounts, and in first-rate formulations. My patients get great results from the products—I see the evidence in my office every day.

The LANCER$_x$ line is not inexpensive (although compared to advanced procedures or plastic surgery, it's reasonable!), so it may not be for everyone. There are good products out there for every budget, as long as you buy wisely. I'll talk more about how to shop for products beginning on page 162, but the specifics I give following the descriptions of each skin care step will also help you find products right for your skin and your budget.

Keep in mind, too, that though products are important, just the sequencing of this anti-aging method is going to do a lot for your skin. Nighttime steps 1 and 2 increase circulation and promote cell turnover as well as clear the path for step 3: delivery of beneficial nutrients. These are the three critical steps. It's not necessary (or recommended for most people) to polish twice a day, so in the morning your third step is applying sunscreen. Sunscreen doesn't change the behavior of the skin the way the other steps do, but it *prevents* damage, which is just as important as repairing damage.

While these steps target aging and are great for treating acne as well, I've frequently seen them repair skin that once seemed irrevocably damaged. About a year ago, a patient of mixed ancestry came to see me. She was part Hawaiian and part Middle Eastern. I was taken aback when I first saw her: she had big black circles around her eyes like a raccoon. "Okay, you've got my attention," I said. "What's the story?"

The patient, who was only thirty-two, had noticed a few sun spots on her face and went to see her aesthetician. She gave her some lightening cream, which caused a terrible red and prickly rash that, when it finally went away, left more spots. She went to another facial spa (a so-called medispa), where something called a "soft light" laser treatment was used over her entire face with the aim of remedying the situation. That's when the raccoon circles surfaced. When I heard that part of the story, I wasn't surprised. Her type of skin is vulnerable to damage from lasers and other therapeutic light sources, a topic I'll talk about in more depth beginning on page 181. The inflammation caused by the "soft light" laser created scarring, which gave my patient the rings around her eyes. It took about seven months, but we were able to reverse it — strictly with the three basic steps I'm recommending to you.

These steps, which I outline below, are important to do every day. Don't slack off! Consistency is key. No matter how tired you are, don't fall into bed without performing your skin care routine first. Your skin repairs itself while you sleep; just imagine it trying to do so with all kinds of pollutants, dead cells, and oil in its way.

Polishing

Most people call this step exfoliation, but I like to call it polishing because the word gives you a good visual image of what you're going to accomplish: removing the sludge (dead skin cells) to reveal fresher, smoother skin. Think of it as taking the tarnish off silver. There are two types of polishers: mechanical exfoliants, which can be anything from a loofah or rough washcloth to a scrub with tiny grains or crystals that rub off dead cells, and chemical exfoliants made of enzyme-based ingredients from plants such as pineapple and papaya that dissolve dead cells. I happen to think that a combination of both tiny scrubbers and enzymes works best. Loofahs and washcloths aren't as efficient, and they can harbor bacteria unless you wash them thoroughly after every use.

When you remove the top layer of dead skin cells, you're not removing all of the stratum corneum (which you'll remember is made up entirely of tightly knit dead cells), but you are removing the dysfunctional cells that have lingered on top too long, causing the skin to look dull and flaky. As those cells are swept away, the layers below get the message to create new skin cells, helping to accelerate cell turnover and bring forth fresh cells. Remember, too, that removing those cells also makes way for the nourishing topical ingredients you're going to add in step 3. Polishing has a few other benefits as well. As you exfoliate, you'll be both increasing the circulation to the skin, giving it an instant glow, and helping to oxygenate the cells, which will increase the effectiveness of reparative proteins and antioxidants.

WHAT TO LOOK FOR: In my own polishing products, I use a combination of mechanical and chemical exfoliants. Most products tend to be one or the other, so faced with a choice, go for the mechanical kind, preferably one made with sea minerals, birch bark, walnut shell, or apricot kernels. Choose a product that will polish your skin without abrading it. The "scrubbers" should be superfine and the product emollient enough to feel comfortable on your skin — that's the mark of high-quality chemistry.

If you prefer to use the type of exfoliant that dissolves dead cells, look for one with natural exfoliating enzymes such as bromelain (derived from pineapple) or papain (from papaya). A good polisher is worth paying extra for.

Cleansing

If polishing is a little like going into a mine and blowing up the rocks surrounding the gems, cleansing is like bringing in a cart to carry all the debris away — it helps you get rid of everything that you've loosened up by exfoliating. The gems are now exposed. That metaphor aside, you're not going for strip-mining here. The removal process shouldn't leave your skin too dry or irritated. A good cleanser will gently remove makeup, sunscreen, dirt, excess yeast, and bacteria and be oil-dissolving enough to remove sebum and other gunk caught in the pores without leaving a film behind. Yet a cleanser shouldn't be so harsh that it leaves your skin feeling very taut or itchy — which is what soap is likely to do.

WHAT TO LOOK FOR: I've had some patients ask me if you need a different cleanser for your eyelids and the answer is no. You should be able to safely use the same product on your entire face, neck, and chest. What you should be looking for in a cleanser is a product that strikes a balance between clearing the skin of dead cells and debris and leaving some of the skin's natural oils intact. Many companies that make cleansers are afraid of creating a product that is overly drying, so they add humectants (substances that promote water retention) and other moisture-gathering compounds to their formulas, and as a result the products leave a film on the skin. It's a bit like the concept of a combination shampoo and conditioner, cleaning and moisturizing in one fell swoop. It may be convenient, but it isn't ideal.

The moisturizing benefit of this type of cleanser may be fine for people who are acne prone or have rosacea, but for anti-aging purposes, choose a stronger cleanser. Most cosmetic cleansers these days employ synthetic cleansers called syndets, which are pH neutral and don't leave a film on the skin. Soaps, on the other hand, drive fats out of the skin and can leave a residue. Your goal should be to find a cleanser that is pleasant to use, non-irritating, non-inflammatory, and soothing — but thorough. Try it out on the soft, non-sun-exposed skin on the inside of your arm; if the cleanser doesn't cause any redness or irritation, chances are it will be okay for your face, neck, and chest. One surprisingly good option is simple baby shampoo, a gentle but thorough cleanser that you can use on your face as well as on the skin on your body.

Some cleansers have added exfoliating ingredients such as salicylic acid, papaya, pomegranate, or alpha hydroxy acids (see page 168). This can help further refine the stratum corneum and prep the skin for nourishment. Many products will give you information about extras such as exfoliating ingredients on their labels. If you don't find what you're looking for, go on to drugstore or beauty product websites and survey the options. You can often read about product details, including active ingredients.

Nourishing

Although I recommend that you nourish the skin from the inside out—eating right and taking the supplements recommended in chapter 3 will help increase your collagen production and replenish your skin with antioxidants—there is only so much you can influence the skin through diet. Eating all the oranges in the world won't give you the therapeutic amounts of vitamin C you need to restore the health of your skin. Plus, there are compounds we know can improve the skin that you can't get through diet at all. That's where topical nourishment comes in.

Nourishing products shouldn't be confused with moisturizers. Though most of them do help the skin retain moisture, nourishers' main role is to deliver antioxidants, vitamins, and other anti-aging ingredients to the stratum corneum. They can come in many forms, including lotion, cream, or serum formulations. As a general rule, be sure to choose a product that feels and smells good to you. It has to be pleasant to use or you're going to conveniently "forget" to put it on, which will ensure that you get no benefit at all. Just as with exercise, you have to be consistent with skin care, and that means complying with *all three* steps on a regular basis.

WHAT TO LOOK FOR: Some nourishers may be labeled as reparative lotions, some as anti-aging creams, others as anti-wrinkle treatments. What's most important is that a) they have active ingredients (and enough of them) to make the skin behave younger, and b) you like the formulation.

Through research, we've been able to determine that many compounds change the skin. But it's still a somewhat inexact science. We know a lot about retinoids — derivatives of vitamin A that I'll discuss shortly — but the benefits of other ingredients are still somewhat poorly defined. Still, we know that if you open up the doors on the skin, which you effectively do by polishing and cleansing, and allow these ingredients in, they will effect positive changes in your skin, provided they're in sufficient amounts and well formulated.

A beneficial day and nighttime nourisher will contain several therapeutic ingredients, among them *antioxidants*. There are many antioxidants used in skin care products, and one is not necessarily better than the next; they just use different metabolic pathways to protect the skin. The following are some that you should look for.

- *Vitamin C* — Vitamin C helps stop free radicals caused by sun exposure from doing damage and may even provide a barrier to the sun's rays. C also protects the collagen you already have and goads the fibroblasts into producing more. Many products now feature vitamin C as an active ingredient. However, not all C is created equal; some forms are very unstable. Be wary of products that have turned brown; this indicates that the C has oxidized and lost potency. Look for C in the form of L-ascorbic acid, the form the body most easily recognizes and gets the best anti-aging results.

- *Vitamin E* — You'll usually see vitamin E on the ingredients list as alpha tocopherol. Vitamin E, an effective free radical scavenger, is especially good at helping to fight inflammation and keeping the skin moisturized. Bear in mind that vitamin E is also a preservative, used to keep cosmetics from spoiling, so if you see it on the ingredients listing, it doesn't necessarily mean it's there in the amount necessary to make your skin younger. Look for E close to the top of the ingredients list.

- *CoenzymeQ-10 (CoQ-10)* — This antioxidant has a useful ability to regenerate the skin, and the molecule's small size makes it easy to absorb.

Newer to the market is idebenone, a close relative of CoQ-10. Idebenone is believed to work similarly to CoQ-10 in the fight against aging.

- *Coffeeberry, Green Tea Polyphenols, Resveratrol*—These antioxidants are increasingly cropping up in skin care products, and they may have some benefits. Here's the caveat. On a microscopic level and in the lab, these and other antioxidants such as pomegranate, grapeseed extract, licorice, and soy, cause some activity within skin cells. When they're applied to the skin on a real, living being, it's difficult to say if they have much effect. I think they can be helpful if they're used in large enough concentrations, but concentrations in most over-the-counter products are probably too low. Expect minimal benefits.

Besides antioxidants, a good nourishing product may also include peptides/pentapeptides. This group of amino acids has a range of anti-aging effects. Some of them, such as palmitoyl pentapeptide-4, help repair broken capillaries and stimulate GAG synthesis and collagen production. When collagen breaks down, it forms peptides, and the peptides signal the skin to make new collagen. Topical peptides have been shown to do the same. Other peptide ingredients work a little like neurotoxins to relax wrinkles on the skin.

Whichever type of nourisher you choose, keep in mind that it's one of the most important products that you'll use. Don't skimp when it comes to nourishers; it's where you should put your money.

YOUR NEW SKIN CARE ROUTINE

Evening

1. *Polish*—Using an exfoliant, polish the damp skin on your face, neck, and chest area for 60 to 90 seconds or according to the product instructions. Rinse thoroughly with lukewarm water. (*Note: If you're wearing foundation, cleanse first, polish, then cleanse again. There's no need to use*

Modifications for Sensitive Skin

I have about ten patients a day who tell me that they have sensitive skin. Some of them actually do have highly reactive skin; others *think* they do. My point is that sensitive skin is often in the eye of the beholder. The kind of sensitive skin that calls for cautionary measures is skin that burns, stings, has uneven color distribution, is pale and flaky, or is red and flaky in response to any kind of irritant, whether the irritant is wind, sun, altitude and temperature and humidity changes, or ingredients in topical products. People who have genuinely sensitive skin also see changes in response to caffeine, alcohol, and spicy and acidic foods. Stress can send sensitive skin into a tizzy, too.

What generally occurs is that these irritants jar the vascular, nervous, and immune regulatory systems in the skin, causing blood vessels to spasm and dilate. Maintaining a healthy lifestyle—eating well, getting adequate sleep, exercising, and controlling stress—goes a long way toward keeping sensitive skin calm. Sensitive skin also responds best to simple skin care. The more complex the products, the more likely they are to hit a trigger. Always look for products that are free of alcohol, witch hazel, fragrance, and color. When buying a polisher, look for one that has "gentle" on the label.

To adjust the polish-cleanse-nourish method for sensitive skin, start with two gentle products formulated for sensitive skin, one cleanser and one nourishing cream; skip the polisher for now. Cleanse and nourish in the morning and the evening for one week. If everything is nice and peaceful, add in the polisher the second week. Watch your skin carefully. If there is any sign of irritation, pull back to polishing once a week, then see if you can gradually increase it without starting the inflammatory roller coaster.

---

a makeup remover—if your cleanser can get rid of sebum and pollution, it should be able to get rid of all your makeup, even mascara.)

2. *Cleanse*—Massage your face (including your eyelids), neck, and chest with a non-irritating cleanser for one minute. Rinse thoroughly with lukewarm water and pat dry.

3. *Nourish*—Apply a nourishing product with free radical–scavenging antioxidants on your face, neck, and chest.

Morning

1. *Cleanse* — Massage your face (including your eyelids), neck, and chest with a non-irritating cleanser for one minute. Rinse thoroughly with lukewarm water and pat dry.

2. *Nourish* — Apply a nourishing product with free radical–scavenging antioxidants on your face, neck, and chest.

3. *Protect* — Follow with an SPF 30 sunscreen, preferably one that also contains antioxidants.

HOW TO SHOP FOR PRODUCTS

The question most people have about skin care products is "How do you know if you're getting what you're paying for?" Nobody wants to shell out hard-earned cash for anything that doesn't deliver. The truth is it's difficult to know if an expensive product will work better than a less expensive one. I know from my own experience developing LANCER$_x$ that the raw components you purchase to put into an anti-aging product can be expensive. When, say, an anti-aging serum is priced at one hundred dollars, it may have a high concentration of antioxidants, peptides, or other ingredients that have been shown to make skin look more youthful. The greater the volume of these ingredients in a product, the more costly it is to produce and, of course, the more expensive the retail price is going to be. But how do you know for sure that there are therapeutic levels of active ingredients in a hundred-dollar serum? Therein lies the problem. Whether it's a vitamin C cream from a high-end line or a vitamin C cream sold at chain drugstores for one-tenth the price, there really isn't any way to tell exactly what you're getting.

There are, though, some clues. If the product has an ingredients list either on the label or within the packaging, look to see where anti-aging components such as vitamins and antioxidants fall. The farther down the list they are, the weaker the concentration of those ingredients. For the most part, you should not expect low-priced products to contain more than low amounts of active ingredients. There is no way a cosmetics company can pump up the volume of active ingredients and keep prices very low. It's also important to realize that a product's effectiveness depends on more than just the potency of the active ingredients. In order for these ingredients to reach the areas of the epidermis and dermis where they do their work, they require "vehicles"—molecules that encapsulate or otherwise capture the ingredients and deliver them into the skin. Delivery ingredients, too, can be costly.

None of this means that low-priced products aren't helpful—many of them are—but it means you shouldn't expect the parting of the Red Sea (or, more to the point, the return of your face to its high school luster). The bottom line is this: A high-priced product from a reputable company may *indicate* the presence of beneficial concentrations of helpful ingredients and efficient delivery systems, but it's no guarantee. Lower-priced products tend to have lower concentrations of the anti-aging components you need, but can still turn back the clock a little bit—especially if you use the polishing-cleansing-nourishing method of skin care. If you're willing to pay for one or two higher priced items, spend your money on a good nourisher first, a good polisher second. Those are the most important products.

Which brings me to another point about skin care products. There is no one magic ingredient destined to be your personal fountain of youth. Attaining beautiful, youthful skin requires a system, and all the pieces need to be in place. You can't just slap on a cream with coffeeberry or green tea and call it a day. Don't be lulled into the concept that one superduper ingredient is the Holy Grail.

DEFENSE! PROTECTING YOUR SKIN FROM THE SUN

Since my practice is in sunny Southern California, there's nothing I hear more than the lament "I shouldn't have spent so much time in the sun." Well, yes, that's true. A lot of my patients, such as Bob, grew up when the only sunscreen available was the zinc oxide lifeguards used to coat their noses. But what's past is past. Let's talk about now, because we know for sure that UV rays are incredibly damaging, and that they not only accelerate the aging of the skin but also put us at risk for skin cancer. The figures are startling: one in five Americans will develop skin cancer in a lifetime. Not all skin cancers are deadly (though even the milder ones can be disfiguring), but sun exposure also increases the risk of the most serious form of skin cancer, melanoma. According to the Skin Cancer Foundation, melanoma rates are rising, and although melanoma has a good survival rate if you catch it early, the rate of survival falls to 15 percent if the disease advances.

Everyone needs sun protection: people with white skin, people with brown skin, people with black skin. For instance, in a 2010 study, black women living in Florida had a 60 percent higher rate of melanoma than black women living elsewhere. I think the message of this study is clear: no matter what color your skin, you can't afford to shrug off sun protection.

If you haven't yet begun using a sunscreen every day, start now. Here are some sun protection guidelines to go by.

Start with sun avoidance. The best way to avoid sun damage is to stay out of the sun. Seek shade whenever possible, and if you have to be out, try to avoid the hours when the sun is strongest, ten a.m. to four p.m. Wear protective clothing, too. The darker and more tightly woven the clothes, the more protection they'll afford. (Save gauzy whites for summer nights—a white T-shirt only has an SPF of 5.) You can also buy clothing with a built-in SPF, or wash it with a laundry aid such as Sun Guard, which gives clothes a higher SPF.

Be smart about SPFs. A product's SPF refers to how long you can stay out in the sun without burning. For instance, if you typically burn in ten minutes without protection, wearing an SPF 15, you can probably stay in the sun for 150 minutes without burning. But that presupposes a few things. One is that the sunscreen you're wearing is absolutely as intact as it was when you first applied it. Sunscreen degrades and gets rubbed off easily; in fact, after two hours, an SPF 30 drops down to an SPF 15, if not lower.

For ultimate protection, you need to reapply sunscreen every two hours. And what is ultimate protection? With sunscreen it's never 100 percent, no matter how high an SPF you choose, so sun avoidance is really your best defense against UV rays. Always wear an SPF 15 or higher, but also be aware that the numbers top out. An SPF 15 blocks 94 percent of rays; an SPF 30 blocks 97 percent. Thus, an SPF 30 doesn't offer twice the protection of an SPF 15; it just has more active ingredients so more of them may stay on as the sunscreen starts to degrade and rub off. That's helpful, but again, you don't want to be lulled into thinking you can stay in the sun longer than you should.

Choose effective ingredients. The active ingredients in sunscreens fall into two categories. As their name suggests, chemical absorbers — aminobenzoic acid (PABA), avobenzone, ecamsule, and oxybenzone, to name a few — work by absorbing radiation. Physical blockers — the minerals titanium dioxide and zinc oxide — work by reflecting and scattering rays. Because chemical absorbers penetrate the skin, they're more commonly linked to skin irritation. Physical blockers aren't absorbed, which is why they often leave a white sheen (and why they're considered the safest choice for kids). My LANCER$_x$ contains a mix of both types of active ingredients, and some other sunscreens do as well.

What's critical is that you select a product that protects against *both* UVA and UVB rays. As you might remember, short-wave UVBs cause sunburn, which is of course very damaging to the skin. But although long-wave UVAs don't cause a burn, they reach way down to the dermis and wreak havoc on cell DNA. SPF numbers refer *only* to protection against UVB rays, so it's difficult to tell if a product also deflects UVAs based solely on its SPF (the FDA has long been promising to come out with a rating scale for UVAs, but it's yet to materialize). But there are clues. Look for the words "broad spectrum" on the label or check the ingredients list; avobenzone, ecamsule, and zinc oxide give the most extensive UVA coverage.

Consider children's sunscreen. Most sunscreens formulated for young children and babies have just about everything you'd want: they're reasonably priced, have a high SPF, have zinc oxide or other blockers that effectively protect against both UVA and UVB rays, and have fewer chemicals that get into the bloodstream (there's no evidence that the chemicals do harm once they're in there, but we do know that the body absorbs them).

———————

Here are some other tips for choosing and using sunscreen:

- The brand or ingredients in a sunscreen are important, but not quite as important as whether you use it, and you're only going to use it if you like it. If it's not easily applied, or if it feels slimy or smears, toss it and buy another one. Some of the higher-priced sunscreens are also higher-quality sunscreens, meaning that they're formulated not just for protection but for comfort as well. And in the long run they'll save you money. I tell my patients that they'll save themselves a lot of money on lasers and fillers if they just stay out of the sun and protect themselves whenever they are exposed.

- Apply sunscreen every day of the year, all over your body. UV rays penetrate clouds and some of them even penetrate glass, including car windows — the left sides of the faces in this car-centric country are usually five to ten years more aged in appearance than the right (it's the opposite in England). In a perfect world, you'll reapply every two hours. Always reapply after swimming, even if the label says your sunscreen is waterproof.

- Slather on your sunscreen thirty minutes before you go out. That will give the active ingredients time to bind with the skin so they can do their work.

- Don't worry about getting your vitamin D from the sun. You may know that the skin, when exposed to sunlight, manufactures the all-important nutrient vitamin D. There has been some concern that sunscreen pre-

---

Skin Care Mistake #3

Not Applying Enough Sunscreen

Sunscreen is not moisturizer. You have to lay it on thick, and few people do: One study found that most people apply only 25 to 50 percent of the recommended amount. When SPFs are tested in the lab, cosmetic scientists layer the cream on uniformly and heavily — a lot thicker than most people do at the beach. The recommended amount to cover an adult body is one ounce (think shot glass). In other words, you've got to really glob it on so that it looks white (your skin will absorb it within a few minutes, so don't worry about the aesthetics). If you're spending days outdoors and not using up a tube of sunscreen in about two days, you're not using enough.

---

vents the production of vitamin D and, indeed, many people don't get enough D — there seems to be an epidemic of vitamin D deficiencies in this country and it's now been linked to everything from cancer to autoimmune diseases like rheumatoid arthritis and Crohn's disease. It doesn't make sense to expose yourself to cancer-causing rays to increase your body's production of vitamin D so, if you're deficient, look to your diet or a vitamin D supplement to make up the difference. See page 127 for more information on vitamin D.

- Be advised that indoor tanning isn't safer than outdoor sun exposure. You can still get a burn, and studies have shown that people who use tanning beds are at higher risk for melanoma than nonusers.

HELP FOR DEEPER LINES AND WRINKLES

If, for whatever reason — maybe you don't have genetics on your side or were a sun worshipper in your earlier years, or a smoker — you have deep lines and wrinkles, you may need to add an extra step or two to your routine to get the results you want. You can benefit from going the extra mile, but not necessarily the extra ten miles. In most cases, simple is always better. Slapping fifteen different products on your skin every day won't make it superior — it will only take you more time (not to mention cost you more money).

The best way to take your skin care routine to the next level is to add either an alpha hydroxy acid (AHA) or a retinoid product — or both — to your arsenal. There are lots of anti-aging ingredients out there, but these two types of interventions have the best track record.

Alpha hydroxy acids. AHAs, as they're commonly known, have exfoliating capabilities. They dissolve the lipids (the "mortar," as you'll remember from my earlier anatomy lesson) that hold together the dead cells in the stratum corneum. As they exfoliate, AHAs also get skin cell turnover back on track. For some people, polishing alone doesn't clear the skin well enough to stimulate accelerated cell turnover.

Among the AHAs, glycolic acid (made from sugar cane) has the smallest molecules, so it penetrates quickest and deepest; however, other AHAs can be effective, too. Lactic acid (from milk), malic acid (from apples), and tartaric acid (from grapes) are AHAs that you will likely also find in reparative creams, cleansers, and other skin care products. AHAs are also used in high concentrations in in-office face peels.

The results you'll get from using an AHA product depend on the concentration of the acid. Most over-the-counter products have fairly low concentrations — about .5 to 1 or 2 percent — but they smooth the skin somewhat. You can also buy products that have 5 to 10 percent concentrations of AHAs, and they do more, helping to lighten age spots and get rid of fine lines. (I have an over-the-counter 10 percent glycolic acid product at lancerskincare.com.) Higher concentrations of AHAs are generally used in peels that need to be supervised by a physician (see page 181).

What's critical to an AHA product's effectiveness is the way it's been formulated. AHAs can be hard on the skin — they sting — so they must be buffered or toned down with other ingredients. Too much buffering negates the power of the AHA, so it's a delicate balance. How well the manufacturer walked that line, though, is hard to judge from the label. Choose a product from a reputable company and give it a month or so to see if it works. You will undoubtedly have some stinging or tingling at first (that tells you that the AHAs are having some effect), but it will likely go away as your skin becomes accustomed to the product. While it's okay for your complexion to turn a light pink, if there is real redness and swelling along with the stinging, it's a sign that the product is too irritating to your skin and you may need to try another.

Alpha hydroxy acids can be used either in the morning or at night. If you use an AHA product in the morning, apply it before your sunscreen and nourisher. If you use it at night, apply after cleansing.

Retinoids. Retinoids, synthetic versions of vitamin A, are one of the greatest discoveries of cosmetic science. They really work to reverse years of sun and environmental damage to the skin. In some ways, they're similar to alpha hydroxy acids — they help slough off dead cells. But retinoids go further, signaling the skin to produce new collagen and hyaluronic acid. Depending on the strength and type of the retinoid you're using, the skin responds fairly quickly: lines and wrinkles smooth out and the skin tone becomes brighter and more uniform. Retinoids are an effective treatment for acne, too.

Retinoids come in different forms. There are several prescription-only creams — tretinoin (Retin A), taxarotene, and adapalene among them — of varying strengths. These are generally prescribed when the problem affecting the skin originates from the lower sections of the dermis, and are sometimes recommended to treat acne, rosacea, and discoloration of the skin. A clinical exam by your dermatologist will tell you if you need a prescription retinoid. He or she can also help you decide which one is right for you and give you samples to try.

You should know, though, that there is a downside to retinoids. While your skin will generally adjust to them, they can be very irritating, so it's imperative to work with your dermatologist to figure out the best formulation for you. You may need to start with a lower-strength product. Retinoids also make the skin more sensitive to the sun and to environmental factors such as altitude; this is the reason they are best applied before bed (though you still need to avoid sun exposure as much as possible). When you're using a prescription retinoid, be careful about the other products you're using. A cleanser or toner that never irritated before may suddenly make your skin red and flaky. If you're also using an alpha hydroxy acid, use the AHA in the morning and the retinoid product at night. If for some reason you can't apply the AHA in the morning, apply the AHA Monday, Wednesday, and Friday nights and the retinoid Tuesday, Thursday, and Saturday nights. It's important to get a group of products that all work well together so that you can continue to have a good skin hygiene program.

Many over-the-counter products now contain retinol, retinal, and other forms of retinoids. I, for instance, use retinol in my AM/PM Nourishing Treatment and Fortified Moisturizer. Over-the-counter retinoids are alternative versions of the prescription-strength retinoids, and they can still make a difference in your skin when used regularly. They are much less irritating, too, so it's something to consider if you have particularly sensitive skin. But even if you don't have sensitive skin, OTC versions are a good place to start. Look for retinol/retinal products that also contain anti-inflammatory ingredients such as green tea polyphenols.

If you're using an over-the-counter product for twenty-one days and don't see improvement, talk to your dermatologist about the possibility of a prescription retinoid. Prescription retinoids are considerably stronger than the OTC counterparts, and they significantly smooth and brighten skin while also making it more even in tone. Whether you're using a prescription or over-the-counter retinoid, check with your doctor before taking any supplements that contain vitamin A, which can be harmful at high levels.

Here are two problems that can be addressed by supplementing your regular routine with alpha hydroxy acids or a retinoid (or both), along with a few other therapeutic products.

FOR DEEP LINES

- At night, after cleansing as you normally would, use a nourisher or separate product containing *coenzymeQ-10* (see page 159 for more on coenzymeQ-10). If you use a separate coenzymeQ-10 product, use that first, then apply your nourisher, and finally smooth on a *10 percent glycolic acid cream.*

Skin Care Mistake #4

Relying Only on "Natural" Products

Natural may be "in" and sound good, but the fact is, these products hardly ever deliver on their promises (besides the fact that "natural" is a nebulous term that could mean virtually anything—in skin care products, the same goes for "organic"). Cosmetic science has made some incredible breakthroughs in the past few years, and it's only the tip of the iceberg. If you're devoted to using only natural products, you're going to miss out! This isn't to say that there is no use for natural ingredients. For instance, many useful antioxidants are from natural sources such as grapes, papaya, and tea. However, products that are made solely from natural ingredients tend to leave gaps in the treatment. Look for products that have medical results to show for themselves and produce pharmaceutical-grade activity, yet have over-the-counter availability. Those are the products that will truly change, correct, and improve your skin. Strive to look natural, not cling to natural products.

- In the morning, put on a collagen-boosting *vitamin C–rich product* after cleansing (if you're using a toner to deal with acne, apply it after the toner). Vitamin C creams can sting a bit, particularly under certain conditions (such as high altitude). If the stinging is too intense, cut back to every other day until your skin adapts.

FOR EXTENSIVE SUN DAMAGE

- In the evening, apply a *retinol cream* before you put on your nourishing product. Sun damage puts you at risk for skin cancer, so make certain that you see your dermatologist every four to six months for checkups. Practice sun avoidance and use a sunscreen daily without fail.

SOLVING SPECIAL PROBLEMS

Sometimes the polish-cleanse-nourish method isn't enough or needs to be altered if you have a particular skin problem. Here are additional steps to take for special needs.

ACNE

- Cleanse with a cleanser made specifically for acne, such as LANCER$_x$ Exfoliating Blemish Cleanser (cleansers for acne usually contain benzoyl peroxide or salicylic acid), then follow with a *nondrying toner* (without alcohol or witch hazel) to gently remove excess oil. Note: If you have sensitive skin, some cleansers made for acne sufferers may be too harsh for you. Some people who have acne believe that the drier the skin, the better. That's not true. Dry out your stratum corneum too much and it sends a signal down below to produce more oil. Watch your results, and if the product isn't working, move on.

- Follow with a *redness relief product* that contains soothing ingredients such as licorice root, bisbolol (made from chamomile), and sodium hyaluronate.

ROSACEA

- Twice daily, use a soothing, *nondrying toner* (see above) after cleansing, but only if you have oily, red, inflamed rosacea. Skip the toner if you have the dry form of rosacea.

- After cleansing (if you have the dry type of rosacea) or toning (if you have the oily kind), use a *redness relief product* (see above).

SEVERE DRYNESS

- In the evening, use a *rosewater spray* to hydrate and calm inflammation, followed by a *nighttime moisturizer* fortified with vitamins and proteins after applying your nourisher. Grapeseed oil (the kind you can buy in the grocery store) is a good inexpensive moisturizer. A costlier, but extremely effective moisturizer is Bulgarian rose oil (see lancerskincare.com).

CREPE-Y SKIN OR DRYNESS AROUND THE EYE

- Put on an *eye cream* after your nighttime nourishing step. The product should have everything your nourishing cream has, but be lightweight, have lower concentrations, and be formulated specifically for the eyes. Grapeseed oil, the kind traditionally used for cooking, also works as an eye cream. Apply the cream from just under your eyebrow down along the top eyelid, then under the eye all the way up to where the bottom lashes begin.

HYPERPIGMENTATION

- At night, before you nourish, use a product specifically designed to lighten pigment and that contains properly formulated *hydroquinone.* The most common causes of skin discoloration are sun damage, inflammation from some kind of injury, and medication. Other ingredients such as niacinamide, malic, pyruvic, and lactic acids can contribute to partial improvement, but hydroquinone works best. Even though hydroquinone is sold over the counter, it's controversial, so talk to your dermatologist about it before you give it a try.

GIVE YOUR NEW ROUTINE SOME TIME

Say you've never done much more to your skin than wash it with soap and water and slather on a moisturizer. Now you're going to be not only giving it a deep cleaning, but also introducing topical ingredients to your skin that are going to nudge it out of a deep sleep and get it back in gear. Your new routine shouldn't cause you pain, but your skin might suddenly become drier and more sensitive.

After about three or four days, all the junk skin sitting on top will be gone. Those layers of dead cells may have made your complexion look dull but they also kept out a lot of things — irritants as well as any potentially helpful ingredients in products you may have been using. So now that those layers are gone, you've got delicate, newly minted skin; fresh dollar bills that haven't been crinkled up yet.

Here's where patience and a little practicality is a virtue. If you find that your skin is rebelling by becoming tight and dry, cut back on the polish to once every third night, or, if necessary, to as little as once or twice a week until your skin recovers. After about twenty-one to twenty-eight days, you

---

Skin Care Mistake #5

Not Eating Enough Dietary Fat

Fat is higher in calories than other macronutrients, so I can see why you might be trying to avoid it, and certainly, fat should be eaten in moderation. But if you're on a severe reduced-fat diet, you're doing your skin a disservice. Dietary fats, including cholesterol, are instrumental in the production of sebum, the oily substance that helps protect and lubricate the skin. Fat is also used by the body to make estrogen and testosterone. The skin not only produces estrogen and testosterone itself—skin is an endocrine organ—but relies on the sex hormones for optimal functioning.

So do include fat in your diet, but not just any kind of fat. Avoid trans fats (partially hydrogenated oils) and saturated fats (such as those in meat and whole dairy products) and opt instead for mononunsaturated fats such as olive and canola oils and foods such as avocado and nuts. Use the 20 Years Younger Diet recommendations for healthy fat intake as outlined in chapter 3 to guide you.

---

should be able to go back to polishing more often. See how much your skin will tolerate as you gradually up the frequency.

Also bear in mind that you may have to adjust your polishing according to hormonal shifts or travel. If you find your skin is oilier, polish more frequently. If you travel to a high altitude or desert where the air is very dry, scale back. If you're in the humid tropics, you might even need to polish twice a day. One of my goals is to see you get into a regular skin care routine, but don't set yourself on automatic. It's important to really pay attention to your skin so you can give it what it needs when it needs it.

Collagen repair begins immediately when you "injure" the skin, which is what, in a sense, good skin care does. The results come from this repair process, but it can take anywhere from six to eight weeks to see those results. So don't expect to see your skin change overnight. Just hang in there and consistently stick to the polish-cleanse-nourish routine.

ALL-OVER YOUTHFULNESS: BODY, HANDS, AND FEET

When was the last time you looked at your whole, unclothed body in the mirror? I thought so. Rarely do we give a glance to parts of our body other than the face. I've already talked about the importance of caring for your skin from the hairline to the breast line. But we're living in a world where more and more people are revealing parts of their bodies. Shorts, sleeveless dresses, short-sleeve shirts, shorter skirts with no stockings, sandals, and slingback shoes (even in winter). More exposure means the need for more comprehensive skin care. Even if you're relatively modest, you don't want to have the face of someone twenty years younger but the hands and feet of someone past his or her prime.

But perhaps even more than that, I find that people want the skin on their body, and particularly the hands and arms, to *feel* better. They want it to feel softer, smoother, and silkier. That's all possible with some easy skin care steps.

The anatomy of the skin on your body from the collarbone down, including the hands and feet, is dramatically different from the skin on your face. The stratum corneum, epidermis, and dermis are much thicker, and the subcutaneous fat takes on a life of its own depending on how much stored body fat you have. The skin on the body also has a slower metabolism, a more leisurely paced skin cell turnover, and it sheds dead cells at a more measured rate. Oil gland production and hair growth is unhurried, too, and the oil and wax secretions are different. Because everything is in slow motion relative to the behavior of the skin on the face, skin on the body doesn't need the same degree of maintenance—but it still needs maintenance.

Restoring the Skin on the Body

When you ask people how they care for the skin on their body, most say, "Oh, soap and some lotion that smells nice." They don't realize that they can do better while still keeping skin care very simple. It's generally a two-step process. You need a mild, non-detergent body cleanser and a hydrating lotion. Something as basic as Cetaphil's Body Wash and Moisturizing Lotion can do the job. Moisturizing lotions are mostly a matter of taste and need. You may want to use a light one in the summer, a heavier one in the cooler, drier months. What matters most is that you apply it daily after showering while your skin is still slightly damp.

If you have more intense sun damage, excessive dryness, discoloration, tiny bumps on the upper arms (called keratosis pilaris), rough elbows, loose, crepe-y skin on the front of the arms, or other problems, I recommend you take body skin care to the next level. Here are the steps to add:

- *Polish.* Use an *exfoliating body scrub* in the shower on an as-needed basis. You may, for instance, use it on the backs of your arms, elbows, knees, and lower legs two times a week but use it on the rest of your body only once a week. Look for a scrub with tiny scrubbers that also contains anti-inflammatory antioxidants (I like green tea and use it in the LANCER$_x$ Body Buff product).

- *Step up moisturizing.* Swap your regular lotion for an *alpha hydroxy acid moisturizer* that contains glycolic or lactic acid, especially if you have very dry skin.

Give Your Hands More TLC

Because they're exposed more than other parts of the body (sometimes even more than the face and neck), the hands can get considerable environmental and sun damage. Over the years, that results in a depreciation of color and texture and the appearance of fine lines, sun spots, and crepe-y skin. Intrinsic changes alter the hands, too. Just like the face, the hands lose fat and the deficit of volume makes them look old and scrawny.

Hand repair does have its limits, but you can do a lot to restore the supple nature of the skin on your hands by decreasing dryness and the fissures that make them feel rough. You can also improve the color of the hands and soften sun spots. It takes these two steps:

Skin Care Mistake #6

Reusing Loofahs and Cleansing Cloths Without Washing Them

Using a loofah, a washcloth, or a coarse-textured Japanese cloth can help exfoliate your skin. However, how often do you wash yours? You need to wash it after every use; otherwise all those old dead skin cells you're removing will cling to the cloth, presenting a nice banquet for bacteria. When you go to use it again, you're increasing your risk of infection. Make sure to wash yours regularly!

- *Polish.* Use an *exfoliating body scrub* on your hands two times a week.

- *Moisturize.* Once a day, use an *alpha hydroxy acid moisturizer* that contains glycolic or lactic acid.

If you have significant sun damage on your hands, I'm afraid that even a good skin care routine won't repair it. You need to look into peels and lasers. Likewise, skin care can't repair volume loss. For that you may want to talk to your dermatologist about fillers.

Fixing Your Feet

The soles of the feet, like the palms of the hands, have a very thick stratum corneum. They develop a callused covering for protection, which isn't much of a problem on the palms, but it can get very dry and cracked on the feet, especially as you get older. The way to deal with it is fairly simple. Apply a glycolic acid foot cream daily for two or three days, then once or twice a week after that as needed. Alpha hydroxy acid creams for the feet are different from the ones you use on your face. The AHA percentages are sometimes lower than those that might be used in a cosmetic peel, yet because they have a different pH, they're able to deeply exfoliate the callused skin on the feet.

Use the glycolic cream after showering. Pat your feet dry, then massage a light layer of the cream all over the bottom of the foot, including in between the toes and anywhere else that is cracked and callused. A good cream will work well without any additional help from a pumice stone or other scrubber.

Anti-Aging Nail Care

As the nails age, they grow more slowly and can become dull and brittle. Eventually, they can become very thick and more curved, too. So you can see why good manicures and pedicures are an important anti-aging strategy. *Good* is the key word. The risk of infection from unclean nail care facilities is high — I have one patient who still hasn't recovered from a life-threatening infection he got from a manicure — so you have to use caution.

Conservative trimming of the nails will keep them clean and smooth, and keeping the cuticles gently pushed back can help prevent infection. The Rolls Royce approach to nail care is to buy your own instruments (such as clippers, cuticle pushers, nail brushes, and emery boards) and have a manicurist come to your home. That way you avoid any potential bacterial outbreaks in a salon. The more affordable and cost-effective approach is to bring your own tools to the salon and ask the manicurist to use them. That way, you're in charge of keeping things clean (up to a point). Whenever you get home from a manicure and pedicure, take a shower and wash your hands and feet thoroughly. That will reduce the potential of anything you picked up at the salon causing an infection.

WHEN YOU NEED A MORE AGGRESSIVE APPROACH

When you care for your skin properly and it begins looking refreshed and radiant, any thought you might have once had about plastic surgery or dermatologist office touch-ups may disappear. Some people, of course, want more, and some people need more. When they do, and after I've had them try alpha hydroxy acids or retinoids, I offer them a conservative, progressive approach to smoothing out lines and wrinkles, replacing volume, improving skin texture, and doing away with sun and age spots.

These anti-aging upgrades, I might add, can all be done without plastic surgery, a message that seems to be getting across. In the last few years, the number of plastic surgery procedures has dropped while the number of non-surgical treatments has increased—and I don't think it's completely due to the economy. For one thing, the innovations in injectables and laser procedures have made these treatments the top choice of men and women seeking to look more naturally youthful. Erase for a moment the picture in your mind of expressionless faces and freakishly inflated lips. When you see a skilled board-certified dermatologist, those aren't likely to be your results. Instead, peels, injectables, and laser procedures—*coupled with good skin care*—can simply make you look healthy and refreshed.

Plastic surgery has its place, and in my opinion it's best used to repair something that has been damaged or is misshapen. Obviously, the shape of someone's nose or asymmetric breasts will not respond to topical treatments. The downside of relying on dramatic aesthetic measures such as face-lifts, brow-lifts, and eyelid surgery is that no matter how well done the procedure is, your face won't match the rest of you. That's another reason I believe that more people are pursuing less invasive interventions. When you opt for the surgical blade, it's often like remodeling the kitchen but leaving the rest of the house looking outdated. But the head-to-toe extreme makeover is not what most people want (or should have).

The menu of anti-aging touch-ups available continues to grow, with some options falling out of fashion as other, more sophisticated treatments take their place. When laser treatments and peels first became popular, they were quite severe—a controlled burn that required major recovery time. But few dermatologists use those drastic procedures anymore. Whereas those treatments worked by triggering a major healing response, many of the treatments we use now are more like tickling: They trigger a natural restoration of the skin that results in an increase in volume and firmness and a healthier tone. These procedures wake up the machinery. Instead of walking out of your doctor's office looking like you were in a house fire, you might be a little pink (there can also be some very mild bruising), but you can go out to dinner that night with minimal makeup.

Each type of treatment has many variations. There are, for instance, dozens of different types of lasers. You'll need to discuss the specifics with your dermatologist—your, I stress, board-certified dermatologist. I am a board-certified dermatologist, which means that along with my regular medical training, I completed a three-year residency in dermatology and passed a test administered by the American Board of Dermatology. Of course I'm going to recommend that you see a board-certified dermatologist for injections, laser procedures, and anything else involving diagnosis and treatment of medical, surgical, and cosmetic concerns of the skin, hair, and nails. This is not just me being territorial. Every day in my office I see what happens when patients receive treatments from people who are not qualified or experienced in giving them. Not only do people get overfilled or treated with the wrong kind of laser, but the person treating them often misses more serious problems. Do your homework. The American Academy of Dermatology can help you find a board-certified dermatologist in your area (www.aad.org/findaderm). For more on who should and shouldn't treat you, you can also go to my website www.lancerskincare.com.

When someone needs more than skin care to address aging, I have him or her try the least invasive procedure first, and then we go from there. Here's what I believe is a good progression.

First Stop: Microdermabrasion

Microdermabrasion is a technique that "sands" the superficial layers of the skin. Dermabrasion is a similar technique, but it causes much greater wounding and has a longer healing process. In most cases, I don't recommend it and certainly not as a first stop. Microdermabrasion, which is gentler, uses an abrasive wand and a vacuum suction to remove the dead skin cells. It's good for sun-damaged skin, age spots, superficial pigmentation, fine lines and wrinkles, clogged pores, blackheads and whiteheads, and some mild acne scars. The neck and chest can also be treated to blend the skin and remove any sun damage found in that area. The procedure takes only about a half hour, and there's little or no healing time.

Second Stop: Chemical Peels

Before a patient tries lasers or injectables, I almost always recommend a chemical peel first. Peels are like an extra-effective polish and cleanse session: they deeply exfoliate the stratum corneum to refresh the skin, smooth lines, and lighten brown spots. They can also be used to remove precancerous lesions. Peels involve the application of a liquid or paste. They can be of varying strengths; some use alpha hydroxy acid solutions, some a mix of acids. The skin generally responds by peeling, the same way it does after a sunburn, and it may take a week or ten days to heal. Some peels — phenol peels, for example — strip the skin so thoroughly that they can be painful and require weeks of healing time. These typically aren't done anymore.

The effects of peels can last from one to several months. You can have them done solely on your eyelids, or section by section, all over your body. If you're having a peel on your face, it's usually a good idea to do your neck and chest, too, so there isn't a disconnect between what's above and what's below the chin.

While not all skin care treatments are recommended for every color skin, all skin colors can handle some form of chemical peel. Your dermatologist can advise you on what type of anti-aging peel will remedy your particular concern. Some are best for acne, some vanquish blotchiness, and others can minimize wrinkles. In my office we typically combine peels with microdermabrasion. Polishing the skin first lets us apply the peel to a primed canvas (so to speak), setting the stage for a clean, smooth, and more predictable response.

Third Stop: Lasers

The next step along the touch-up continuum is laser resurfacing. Einstein laid the groundwork for the invention of lasers (light amplification by the stimulated emission of radiation) — that's how far back they go. In 1963, they became medical grade, and I've been using them myself since the 1970s. But today's lasers are nothing like the ones we used back then, when there were only two suitable for dermatological use, both of which burned the skin and required major recovery time. Today's lasers are highly refined, and the skin heals quickly after most treatments if properly done on well-primed skin. (I can't overemphasize the need for skin conditioning before a procedure!)

Lasers and other energy-based treatments generally work by triggering a healing response that leaves skin softer, smoother, and tighter. But that's really a generalization, because there are so many energy-based treatments available now and they all have their unique means of reaching a particular end. There are, for instance, treatments for brown, blotchy discolorations on the skin. Some lasers are used for correcting fine lines, scars, or pore enlargement. Some tone or tighten skin. Others remove hair or broken blood vessels. There are lasers that specialize in removing tattoos as well as permanent eyebrow and lip lines. There are even liposculpting lasers that work from the inside (this is an invasive procedure) to tighten and contract the skin. And not all energy-based treatments use lasers. Other technologies include infrared light, which uses heat (versus light) to tighten loose skin; intense pulsed light (IPL), a tool effective for redness, rosacea, and excess melanin, and for improving color and pore size; radiofrequency, which helps produce new collagen; and light-emitting diode (LED), which helps with acne, wrinkling, and pigmentation.

If you've tried a chemical peel and want to go to the next step, start with a nonablative laser treatment. Also called nonwounding lasers, these are best at making minor corrections on the skin, firming and improving tone and texture. They work beneath the top layers of the skin to trigger collagen production and other repair mechanisms. Another option is fractional resurfacing, which delivers a series of microscopic, closely spaced laser spots to the skin while simultaneously preserving the normal healthy skin between those spots. This is a good option for improving fine lines, wrinkles, brown pigmentation, sun spots, age spots, and acne scarring. And because the laser preserves the healthy skin, the healing is rapid. The entire face can be treated in about forty-five minutes with very little discomfort; there's no need for pain medication and no significant downtime. Both types of laser techniques require several sessions spaced three to four weeks apart.

The most invasive type of lasers are called ablative. Because they go deep and effectively vaporize the top layer of the skin, they create dramatic results in only one treatment — you get more bang for your buck. However, these lasers require significant finesse and there's more healing time (seven to ten weeks).

Laser treatments are not without risk. Some can cause loss of pigment, scarring, or an unattractive change in skin texture. If you have black or brown skin, be sure to go to a dermatologist who is well versed in treating darker ethnicities. And no matter how your skin looks to the naked eye, be certain your doctor also knows your ethnic heritage, especially if it's mixed. In 1998 I introduced a scale that dermatologists can use to predict whether their patients are appropriate candidates for laser treatments. The scale assigns a number, 1 through 5, to each grandparent of the patient. Grandparents who were African get a 5; grandparents from Nordic areas get a 1. The total is then divided by 4 to get the patient's LES (Lancer Ethnicity Scale) score. The lower the score, the lower the risk of scarring and uneven pigmentation after laser treatments. Here are a few other suggestions. Remember: Procedure means risk!

- *Don't get lasered at the mall.* Every day I see scars from laser treatments performed by people who shouldn't be operating the equipment even if there is no law against it. Lasers can be damaging if they're not used properly. Go to a board-certified dermatologist who will perform the treatment him- or herself, preferably one with years of experience and many different lasers (that way there's a greater chance that he or she will use the absolute best tool for the job).

- *Be prepared for the cost.* Laser treatments can run into the thousands of dollars.

- *Know the likelihood of success.* Do lasers work for everybody? No, although they have a very good record. Patients tend to fare better if their skin has good elasticity and they are relatively thin. Talk to your doctor about what you can reasonably expect from the treatment. Realistic expectations are a must.

Last Stop: Injectables

Injections of compounds that plump up or freeze wrinkles and firm slack skin should be last on your list of interventions. The concept of injecting something into the body to increase volume seems relatively new, but even a hundred years ago, fat fillers were used to help in recovery from battle wounds. There are also reports in the medical literature going way back of people injecting themselves with oil and waxes.

The first big commercially used dermatologic filler was silicon, and some doctors are still using it today. There's no law against it, but there probably should be. Unlike other injectables, silicon doesn't dissolve, so even if the initial injection doesn't trigger an inflammatory immune response, eventually the immune system will wake up and the body will start to wall off the silicon, creating rock-hard tissue and other problems. Don't go there — it's not worth it.

Modern fillers and wrinkle-freezers eventually dissolve. Fillers not only fill the space where collagen and fat used to be, but also stimulate a controlled response in the skin (not an unpredictable one as happens with silicone) that triggers collagen production, creates volume, and attracts water to the skin. Depending on which type of injectable you choose, they're good for improving fine lines and wrinkles, making lips fuller, filling hollow cheeks, and plumping up deep folds. Injectables tend to be used around the mouth, eyes, cheek, jaw, brow, and bridge of the nose. But they can be used anywhere there is tissue volume loss (hands, breast, buttocks, for instance).

Wrinkle-freezers, also known as neurotoxins, work by blocking the nerve receptors on the muscle to inhibit wrinkle formation. Think of it this way. Water in a cup ripples when you tap it; frozen water doesn't. It sounds like it will feel weird, but there's no odd sensation. After treatment, patients can still frown and smile normally, but when they do, the crinkles around their eyes and forehead are greatly diminished. The effects last about four months.

Most patients get neurotoxin injections to address crow's feet and forehead lines, but you don't want a total elimination of lines and faults in the

> ## *How Much Do I Need?*
>
> As a general rule, tell your doctor how much of a change you want to see as a result of an injectable treatment. Next, ask him how much of a change he thinks you should pursue. Average out these two — then cut the sum in half. You can always go back and get more, which may be inconvenient, but far better than walking away from the office looking overplumped or too frozen. Too much of a filler can distend the skin and result in a very unnatural look that becomes permanent because the skin has been overstretched. Too much of a neurotoxin can obliterate your facial expressions. The goal is to look younger, not like you're in a coma! One of my patients, who comes to see me all the way from the East Coast, always says, "Don't give me my money's worth." In other words, don't overfill. It's a smart request.

skin. You want a *reduction;* otherwise you'll look so altered that it will be obvious from a hundred yards away that you've had Botox. You want to look fresh and radiant, not "fixed."

Your dermatologist can help you decide which brand-name filler or freezer best meets your needs. Some fillers are made from compounds natural to the body like collagen and hyaluronic acid, while others are made from synthetics. Botox is the most famous neurotoxin, but there are others on the market, too.

Injectables are relatively reasonable in price — they start at a few hundred dollars — but they require somewhat of a commitment on your part. While it varies from person to person, you'll probably need filler injections about twice a year, sometimes more often depending on what's used. That's not only because the fillers don't last, but also because the clock keeps ticking, meaning you'll lose more volume and have more to fill as time goes on. Most people are pleased when they see their faces looking twenty years younger, but some people get a little too pleased. They want more and they begin to get a distorted idea of what looks attractive. That's when you start seeing frozen foreheads and platypus lips, a sign that both the patient and the physician have lost their sense of proportion and artistry. It's also a sign that injections have become an unhealthy addiction.

It's a dangerous addiction, because even though most fillers and wrinkle-freezers eventually dissipate, there's still a chance of permanent damage. Think about a balloon. If you keep filling it up, it begins to lose its original shape when the air is gone. That's what happens to the face or any part of the body if you're not conservative with fillers. In the case of injectables, less is more. Before you embark on treatment, make sure that you and your dermatologist agree on appropriate goals.

Order from the Menu Sensibly

The beauty buffet is wide, but I encourage you to use restraint. You'll hear a lot about all the different procedures that can make you look younger, but there's no need to jump on the bandwagon at every turn. When you take good care of your skin, you may not need to spend a lot of money or take risks to turn back the clock. Remember you're not just going for the illusion of youth; you want your skin to *act* younger.

Think, too, about how a skin care regimen can keep your complexion youthful and vibrant for life. It's something you can always do by yourself — you don't have to worry about a procedure wearing off and going through the whole thing again...and again...and again. Skin care is easy, it's quick, it's relatively inexpensive, and *you* are in the driver's seat.

CHAPTER 5

Rejuvenating Sleep

By Ronald L. Kotler, MD, DABSM

A MAN, NINETY YEARS OLD, was asked to what he attributed his longevity. "I reckon," he said with a twinkle in his eye, "it's because most nights I went to bed and slept when I should have sat up and worried." That little tale, true or not, was a favorite of Dorothea Kent, an actress who hit her prime in the 1930s. Kent frequently played the quintessential dumb blonde, but she was smart if she thought that there was an association between long life and sleep. In fact, she got it exactly right.

Anyone can tell you that getting a good night's sleep makes you look and feel better, but now we also know for certain that lack of sleep predisposes you to several life-shortening diseases. Research shows, for instance, that it doesn't take long for someone with a sleep deficit to begin developing problems related to obesity. Not only does the body's ability to process sugar become impaired, but the hormone that makes you hungry increases and the one that tells you you're full decreases, setting the stage for ample weight gain. There's also evidence that getting less than six hours of sleep per night can increase your risk of heart disease, stroke, and depression. Finnish researchers have even found that getting less than seven hours of sleep increases the risk of early death by 26 percent in men and 21 percent in women.

Sleep is like the air we breathe; we need it to be healthy in virtually every way, as well as to be safe. Skimping on the proverbial forty winks can lead to serious injury, sometimes even premature death. The National High-way Traffic Safety Administration estimates that each year more than 100,000 people crash on the highways because of drowsy driving. Many are killed or permanently injured.

So getting enough sleep doesn't just make you look and feel better — it's powerful preventive medicine. Just as you eat healthfully and exercise to improve and maintain your well-being, it's essential to follow a regimen that promotes adequate and restful sleep.

A lot happens while you're sleeping. During the day when you're active, your energy resources are directed toward maintaining your body. But at night, the construction crew gets to work. It's thought that the body regener-ates bone and muscle as you sleep while also repairing and synthesizing pro-teins that are critical to every part of the body, from the immune system to the skin. Regeneration of connections in the brain and consolidation of memories and emotions are also believed to take place during sleep, undoubt-edly one reason cognition is better when you're well rested.

One of the biggest myths is that you need less sleep as you get older. That's simply not true. In general, adults past the age of about eighteen need seven to nine hours of sleep. It's thought that exactly how much each indi-vidual needs is genetically determined, and it's important to figure out exactly what works for you. Aim for the amount of sleep that makes you feel refreshed throughout the day. While there are rare individuals known as "short sleepers" who can get by with fewer hours of nightly slumber, most people who sleep less than seven hours per night build up a sleep debt and have trouble staying awake during the afternoon. This is your body's way of telling you not to sacrifice your much-needed sleep.

Interestingly, there is evidence that regularly sleeping *more* than nine hours may put you at risk for life-threatening diseases such as diabetes and obesity. But this isn't nearly as big a problem as not getting enough sleep, particularly as you get older. As you age, you *need* just as much sleep but it becomes increasingly difficult to *get* as much sleep. Age-related changes in the sleep cycle diminish the amount of deep, restorative slumber you experi-ence each night, which not only affects the quality of your sleep but also makes it harder to sleep through the night without waking. Waking wouldn't be so bad if you could fall immediately back to sleep; however, it's common for people to have trouble dozing off again. People with insomnia often find themselves tossing and turning, worrying about not getting enough sleep — a self-perpetuating cycle if there ever was one.

Dire as that sounds, there's actually a lot you can do to compensate for changes in the sleep cycle and improve both the quantity and the quality of your sleep. In chapter 4, Dr. Lancer talked about skin hygiene; here, I'm going to talk about sleep hygiene: healthful practices that help you nod off at night and maintain restorative sleep. Sleep hygiene is actually connected to skin hygiene, just as it's linked to healthy eating, exercise, and other anti-aging topics in this book. When you're well rested, you're going to have the energy and inclination to exercise and cook nutritious meals, as well as be less likely to shrug off your skin care regimen. Your skin is going to look more refreshed, too. Being well rested will also put you in a more positive frame of mind, helping you cope better with youth-sapping stress. Sleep simply gets you operating in high gear.

The tenets of sleep hygiene will make a lot more sense once you understand the different phases of sleep and the biological rhythms that govern them.

AGING AND THE SLEEP CYCLE

Whether or not you're aware of it, your body runs on a clock; several clocks, in fact. An area of the brain called the hypothalamus generates what's known as biorhythms, cyclical patterns that regulate just about every physiological process in the body. The menstrual cycle is an example of a monthly biorhythm; appetite, body temperature, blood pressure — and sleep — are all influenced by daily biorhythms. When we talk about sleep, we refer to its biorhythm as a circadian rhythm (*circa* means "around," *dian* means "day"). The sleep-wake circadian rhythm is determined by a highly complex interaction between light and neurotransmitters in the brain. When it's dark, our bodies are programmed to seek sleep, and when it's light they're programmed to stay awake. Our use of light bulbs to light up our night has skewed things slightly, but when everything is working properly, our bodies are still inclined to follow the sleep-wake schedule we evolved with: on average, sixteen hours of wakefulness and eight hours of sleep.

To stick to this schedule, the body releases chemicals that wake you up with the morning's light and keep you alert for several hours thereafter. Between one and six p.m. — the exact time can vary from person to person — you'll probably feel a dip in energy and maybe even feel like falling asleep. It's so predictable that many countries build a midafternoon break (the siesta) into their day, and if you don't nap you've probably developed some way of coping, perhaps taking a coffee break, visiting the office vending machines, or walking around the block to shake off drowsiness. As the day goes on, you get a second wind, but you also build up what's known as a sleep drive — a desire to sleep that gradually increases as you stay awake. During the evening, further biochemical changes in the body increase the sleep drive until finally, by about eleven p.m. for most people, you want — and need — to go to bed.

The sleep-wake circadian rhythm is an elegant, well-designed system; however, it does change at different times of life. Adolescents and teenagers, for instance, experience a shift that cues them to go to sleep later and wake up later. Aging has an impact on the circadian rhythm, too. It's very common for people ages sixty-five and up to experience the opposite of the adolescent/teenage phenomenon: Their circadian rhythms tell them to go to sleep earlier and wake up earlier.

If you're getting enough high-quality sleep, it doesn't necessarily matter when you go to bed and get up. But other age-related physiological changes can make getting enough high-quality sleep challenging. And what is high-quality sleep? Stage 3 sleep, also known as deep or slow-wave sleep.

When you're asleep, your brain exists in one of two states: non-REM sleep or REM sleep. REM stands for rapid eye movement and it describes the stage of sleep in which most dreaming occurs. The complete cycle of non-REM and REM sleep takes about ninety minutes, then starts all over again.

During REM sleep you're virtually immobilized; you might twitch a bit, but you have limited movements in your arms and legs. When you first nod off, you go immediately into non-REM sleep, then you go into REM sleep, toggling between the two so that you go into REM sleep about four to six times per night. The first bout of REM is only one to five minutes long, but REM sleep gets progressively longer through the night so that you're in it an average of eighteen to twenty-two minutes per episode. REM sleep makes up about 20 to 25 percent of an adult's night sleep, and that figure stays pretty constant as you age. The reason that REM sleep is important is not fully understood, but it's believed to contribute to overall emotional and psychological well-being.

Non-REM sleep is the type of sleep you need for repair and restoration of the body. Unlike REM sleep, non-REM sleep changes as you get older, beginning at around age thirty. Non-REM sleep is divided into three stages, 1, 2, and 3. Stages 1 and 2 are the lighter stages of sleep. Stage 3 is known as deep or slow-wave sleep (each phase of sleep has distinctive brain waves that are measurable on high-tech monitors), and it's what you need to feel refreshed in the morning. For some reason that has yet to be discovered, deep sleep diminishes greatly as you age. By the time you reach your seventies and eighties, your slow-wave sleep can be minimal or totally absent. What's more, the slow-wave sleep you do have isn't as deep as it was when you were younger.

The age-related ebb of slow-wave sleep presents a few different problems. With less deep sleep, you spend more time in the lighter stages of sleep, so not only do you get less refreshing sleep, but you're often in a stage from which you can be easily awoken. And because the depth, not just the length, of your deep sleep changes with age, you can be more easily awoken in stage 3 sleep, too. A creak in the floor, the slam of a neighbor's car door, and you're up.

Your vulnerability to being prematurely awakened changes through the years. When my son was about two years old, we took him to a wedding. During the reception, he crawled under the table and fell fast asleep. Despite blasting music and people dancing all around us, he remained in a deep sleep. At age two, he had the luxury of having plenty of stage 3 sleep. Now consider a fifty-four-year-old man, who as an empty nester decides along with his wife that it might be nice to leave their quiet, tree-lined suburban home and spend a few nights a week in the city. On the first night in their little studio apartment, it becomes clear that sleeping is going to be a challenge. The sound of sirens, traffic, people talking and partying in the street — sounds that probably wouldn't have bothered him if he were in his twenties — wake him up repeatedly. Now every time he spends the night in the city, he wears earplugs.

When you become a lighter sleeper, you are susceptible not only to external disturbances (e.g., honking horns and car alarms) but to internal ones as well. So if, like many people as they age, you have some sort of medical condition or complaint, it becomes increasingly likely that pain or discomfort will wake you up. Gastric reflux (otherwise known as heartburn), arthritis, a bum knee or other orthopedic problem, breathlessness from heart or lung disease, hot flashes associated with menopause, prostate issues that create the urge to urinate — any of these can leave you staring at the ceiling at two a.m. And as you get older, you may be more likely to take medications that disturb sleep. Asthma medicines, for instance, can be stimulating. Some antidepressants and heart and blood pressure medications can cause wakefulness, and diuretics can make the urge to urinate hard to ignore.

Good restorative sleep habits are your best defense against disrupted sleep, but there are some conditions that can't be fixed with good sleep practices alone. If you think any of the following three problems might be causing you to lose sleep, it's important to find ways to cure or cope with them as you simultaneously begin implementing the sleep hygiene advice I outline in this chapter.

OBSTRUCTIVE SLEEP APNEA

According to the American Sleep Apnea Association, sleep apnea affects about 12 million Americans, but the vast majority of cases goes undiagnosed. If you have sleep apnea, you might lie down, fall asleep, and progress into stages 1 and 2. Then, just as you're getting ready to descend into deep slow-wave sleep, the muscles in the back of your airway collapse, obstructing breathing. At first this just causes snoring, but as the airway narrows and airflow becomes either partially or fully blocked, the brain responds by sending a powerful message to the airway muscles to open up—and they do. However, the brain's message also triggers the release of catecholamines, stimulating hormones that prepare the body to either fight or flee a potentially harmful situation (the "fight or flight" response). This not only disrupts the normal progression of sleep but also increases the risk of high blood pressure, heart attack, and stroke.

Obstructive sleep apnea can hit at any age, and the likelihood of developing it increases as you get older. Like a lot of areas in the body, the airway muscles can begin to sag as you get older, increasing the risk that when they relax (everyone's airway muscles relax during sleep; it's just a question of how much) they'll block the flow of air. Being overweight makes you more prone to sleep apnea. If you aren't feeling refreshed when you wake up, are feeling extremely fatigued, wake yourself (or your bed partner) up by snoring, or have been witnessed to stop breathing as you sleep, it's essential that you see your physician.

A sleep study is necessary to confirm the diagnosis of obstructive sleep apnea and to determine its severity. During a sleep study, you spend the night at a sleep center, where you're hooked up to various monitoring devices. (Make sure your sleep study is performed at a center accredited by the American Academy of Sleep Medicine—www.aasmnet.org.) If you do have obstructive sleep apnea, the primary treatment is nasal CPAP (continuous positive airway pressure). This is a device that blows air through your nose to the back of your throat and keeps your airway from collapsing while you sleep. Sleep apnea can also be treated by the use of an oral appliance typically made by a dentist, removal of the tonsils, or surgical correction of a deviated nasal septum. If you're overweight, weight loss alone can lead to a dramatic improvement. Depending on the severity of your sleep apnea, your physician may advise you to wear CPAP as you sleep while you work on losing weight.

MENOPAUSE

The most obvious menopausal symptom to disrupt sleep is hot flashes. But you don't have to have hot flashes to suffer from menopausal-related sleep problems. I have seen plenty of patients who were great sleepers all their lives suddenly experience insomnia even though they're not having hot flashes. Fluctuating estrogen and progesterone levels can be wildly disruptive to regular sleep patterns and make it difficult to drift off at night. When a woman has hot flashes to boot, it's a double whammy, with hormonal changes making it hard to *fall* asleep and the hot flashes making it hard to *stay* asleep.

Some women find relief with the help of a light sleeping pill. Hormone replacement therapy is another option, though it's important to discuss the risks with your physician (see page 125 for more on HRT). If you're looking for a natural solution, you might try black cohosh, a Native American herb that can help with hot flashes. Hot flashes can also be less disruptive if you wear very light clothes to bed (there are even special pajamas and nightgowns in "dry" wicking fabrics manufactured for people with night sweats), avoid spicy foods, and use a fan to cool you down.

GASTRIC REFLUX

One of my patients likes to tell me that when he was a teenager he could eat a Philly cheese steak and half a pizza at midnight, go to bed, and sleep like a baby. Now in his fifties, he has to wait four hours from his last bite in the evening before he can go to bed. Otherwise, he lies down and the next thing you know, he's starting to cough and has an acid taste in his mouth — heartburn, the more common name for gastric reflux.

Gastric reflux, which occurs when food and stomach acid come back up into the esophagus, is yet another malady that becomes more common as we age. There are a couple of reasons why. One is that it's not unusual for the tiny hole in the diaphragm that allows the esophagus to connect to the stomach to become defective with age. The hole gets bigger and the stomach pushes up into the chest — it's called a hiatal hernia — allowing the food and acid that should be going south to move north. Gastric reflux can also occur when a little muscle called the esophageal sphincter, which separates the esophagus from the stomach, becomes stretched out. The sphincter usually does a good job of keeping the contents of the stomach from moving back up, but when it's compromised, heartburn happens.

Since gastric reflux is worse when you're reclining, it can make sleep difficult to achieve and maintain. And there can be more serious consequences. I have had patients whose reflux led them to bring up food and acid that then went through their vocal cords and into their lungs while they were sleeping. They ended up in the emergency room at three a.m. with pneumonia. Anything like that, however, is less likely to happen if you take preventive measures. Like my former cheese-steak-and-pizza-eating patient, give yourself a three- or four-hour stretch between your last bite and bedtime. If that's not possible, start your night's slumber in a comfortable chair so you don't lie in bed wide awake because of the discomfort.

You'll be less likely to experience reflux if you shift the bulk of your calories to the earlier part of the day (a good practice regardless) and eat a relatively small dinner made up of low-fat, non-fried foods — meals, in other words, in line with the recommendations in chapter 3. Skip acidic fruits and vegetables, mints, candy, alcohol, and caffeine at night. Use antacids as necessary, but if you're using them every night, you need to see your physician. A doctor can diagnose the cause of the problem and suggest remedies. Some prescription medications such as H_2 blockers and proton pump inhibitors can suppress acid production and be very helpful. If medication doesn't work, discuss surgical options with your physician.

There are other problems beyond these three that can lead to disrupted sleep. Restless legs syndrome, which produces uncomfortable sensations in the legs and a desire to move them, is one. A condition called propriospinal myoclonus, which involves sudden movement that keeps you from falling asleep, night terrors, and sleepwalking are other conditions to see a sleep specialist about.

GETTING A GOOD NIGHT'S SLEEP: AN 11-POINT PLAN

So far, we haven't found a way to shift the balance of light and deep sleep in older people back to its younger and more restful ratio. But we have found that there are many ways to compensate, and if you maintain healthy sleep practices, you can still get all the rejuvenating sleep you need to fight disease and ensure that your body functions in top form regardless of age. The following sleep hygiene tips are tried and true. Check them off your list and you'll raise the odds considerably of getting a good night's sleep. Believe me, you're going to find that they work a whole lot better than counting sheep.

1. Be Consistent

The best way to make certain that you get seven to nine hours of sleep each night is to go to bed and wake up at the same time every day — or close to it. Even if you pride yourself on being a free-spirited, spontaneous kind of person, your body yearns for a regular schedule. A bedtime that zigzags from eleven p.m. one night to three a.m. the next, then back to eleven p.m. — with a corresponding crisscross of wake-up times — throws your system off and can lead to sleep disruption.

When it comes to consistency, I really try to practice what I preach. I get to bed about eleven p.m. weeknights and get up at about seven a.m. On the weekends I might go to bed an hour later and sleep an hour later, but I try not to vary it more than that. Think about what happens when you stay up until two: to get eight hours of sleep in, you don't get up until ten. Maybe you'll try to return to your regular schedule and go to bed at eleven, but because you woke up at ten that morning, you're not tired at eleven, so you stay up a few more hours… You see where I'm going with this. Diverting too far from a regular pattern sets you up for a vicious cycle of insomnia and disturbed sleep.

As part of your consistency plan, try to get outside every morning (or sit by a window) so that you have some exposure to light. Morning is a great time to exercise outdoors. Morning light exposure helps set your clock for the day, helping you to feel tired enough to sleep when bedtime rolls around.

2. Have a Bedtime Routine

Have you ever felt absolutely exhausted, dropped into bed, then had trouble falling asleep? This is a common scenario, because even if you feel tired, your brain needs time to wind down before it can slip into sleep. It's not enough to have a relaxed body; you also need a relaxed brain. Very few people can work on the computer, answer e-mails, or watch TV until eleven p.m., then turn off their brains, roll over, and fall fast asleep. And this is particularly true of people prone to insomnia. One reason it's so difficult to do is because many of the devices we use in the evening involve light, which, as you'll remember, cues the brain to stay awake. It doesn't help that your mind will likely be aroused by what you've been reading or watching, adding another barrier to sleep.

Your first line of defense should be to organize your day in a way that's conducive to helping you slow down in the evening. Take care of all the computer and phone work you need to do earlier in the day, and if you have to have any stressful conversations, make sure you have them well before it's time for bed. Also, create a schedule for yourself that ensures that you don't eat dinner or exercise too close to lights-out (I'll talk more about these in a minute).

Then get into the habit of quieting down in the evening. Dim the lights as the night wears on and give yourself a pre-bed ritual. It might involve straightening up a bit, setting aside things you'll need in the morning, brushing your teeth, flossing, and going through your skin care routine (Dr. Lancer's polish-cleanse-nourish method!). If you have the time and inclination, take a warm bath — it's been shown to help hurry sleep onset. Adding a lavender scent to the water has been proven to be relaxing, too. Reading in bed is another good way to get your brain to ease into sleep. Many people find this to be a very soothing activity, especially if the material isn't too exciting. When you go through the same routine every night, it's going to signal your brain that it's time for sleep. If you have difficulty falling or staying asleep, consider reading in a room other than your bedroom using a low-watt light.

Only use your bed or bedroom for sleep (the exception, as just noted, being reading if it helps you drift off to sleep). If it doesn't lead to a persistent state of arousal, sex is okay, too. Pavlov conditioned dogs to hear a bell and salivate because they associated the bell with food. Our brains react similarly to suggestion. If you condition your brain to see your bed as a place for sleep, as soon as you walk into the bedroom biochemical changes are going to occur that increase the likelihood that you'll fall asleep. Conversely, if you watch TV, work on the computer (or your smart phone), or have upsetting phone conversations with your mother-in-law in the bedroom, your brain is going to associate your bedroom with stimulation. For most people, sex can lead to a state of deep relaxation and help ease you into sleep. But there are some people who have trouble falling asleep after sex. Coordinate the timing of intimacy with your partner so that you can both get a good night's sleep.

3. Empty Your Mind

Stress and anxiety can prevent you from falling asleep by making it hard to slip into that relaxed-brain mode I was just talking about. They can also wake you up in the middle of the night, as anyone who's found himself panicking about mortgage payments at four in the morning can tell you. Before you go to bed (or after you've gone to bed but cannot sleep because your mind's on overdrive), sit quietly in a room other than your bedroom and write down all of the things you need to attend to the next day. Realize, too, that these are things you can't work on right now. You can't call the mortgage company. You can't talk to your boss right now (and don't even think about sending her an e-mail!). You can't discuss the washing machine problem with your soundly sleeping spouse. So write it all down — that will give you some peace of mind, because now you're not going to forget anything tomorrow. Leave the piece of paper in the other room and go to bed.

4. Not Before Bed: Alcohol, Caffeine, Nicotine, a Big Meal

If you need another reason not to smoke besides that it's the absolute worst thing you can do for your health, consider that smoking also interferes with sleep: Nicotine's stimulating effect can keep you up at night. What's more, research suggests that smokers take in less oxygen while they sleep, which may lead to a variety of conditions that can cause premature death.

Caffeine, as you probably already know, is also a stimulant, but what you may not know is that it can stay in your body for as long as fourteen hours. If you're very sensitive to caffeine, avoid coffee, tea, chocolate, and caffeinated sodas for ten or twelve hours before bedtime. It's also a good idea to avoid alcohol in the late afternoon and evening if you typically have trouble sleeping (moderate drinking is okay if it doesn't seem to bother you). Though it initially acts as a sedative, as alcohol is metabolized it has a stimulating effect on the body that may make it hard to fall asleep or may wake you up. Alcohol also exacerbates snoring and sleep apnea. If you must have a nightcap, make it something soothing, such as chamomile tea, or a beverage that contains calcium, such as milk or a yogurt drink. Calcium works as a natural sedative for some people.

Like alcohol, a big meal might make you sleepy at first, but you will suffer for it later. If you try to go to sleep after a big meal, your body is going to be too busy digesting the food to sufficiently move into relaxation mode. Likewise, eating anything high in fat or protein close to bedtime may keep you awake (they take longer to digest than carbohydrates). If you're prone to reflux (see page 194), you also run the risk of ending up with an insomnia-inducing case of heartburn.

To Nap or Not to Nap?

A lot, both pro and con, has been said about napping, so let me clear it up for you. A thirty-minute nap can be very energizing and refreshing and, if you have the time, it's a good way to recharge. Earlier I mentioned that it's common to have an afternoon dip in energy. That dip is going to feel like the Grand Canyon if you're not getting high-quality sleep at night. For some people, a power nap is the perfect remedy.

Discovering whether or not a power nap works for you may take some trial and error. And there are some caveats. If you have insomnia, I don't recommend napping, because it diminishes your sleep drive. When you try to fall asleep later that night, it's going to be rough going. Even if you don't suffer from insomnia, make sure you don't nap too close to dinnertime or for longer than thirty minutes. A long nap or a nap just before or after dinner will probably make it hard for you to drift off to sleep at bedtime.

It's also important to realize that naps are not a substitute for a good night's sleep. A thirty-minute nap isn't enough to give you the deep sleep you need to repair your body and refresh your mind. So while a nap can help you make up some lost sleep, it can't replace healthy nighttime sleep.

---

5. Exercise Often and at the Right Time of Day

Exercise, and cardiovascular exercise in particular, is probably the best natural sleep aid you can find. Regularly getting your heart rate up triggers the release of endorphins and may have a positive effect on serotonin levels, both of which help relieve stress and promote deep, restorative sleep. For those same reasons, exercise also helps lower the risk of depression and one of its side effects: insomnia. Yet to get the sleep benefits of exercise, timing is everything. Vigorous physical activity causes the release of adrenaline, putting your body in an excited state that makes it hard for you to drop off. It also elevates body temperature, another obstacle to falling asleep. Try to get your workout in earlier in the day, or at the latest no closer than three hours before bed. If, however, you're game to do some gentle stretching or a stroll around the block before bed, I'd recommend it. Any movements that help you relax without raising your body temperature can help send you off into dreamland. Just make sure that prior to starting a vigorous exercise program you check with your physician to make sure it is safe to do so. For more on exercise, check out chapter 2.

6. Block Out Stimuli

This is an especially important part of sleep hygiene for anyone in midlife and older. Now that you spend longer amounts of time in the light sleep stages and your deep sleep isn't as deep as it used to be, you need to anticipate noise, movement, and other disruptions that can jolt you awake. Close the drapes, shut your bedroom door, turn off or remove any electronics giving off ambient light — you might even go as far as installing soundproof windows or blackout curtains. An eye mask, earplugs, and some kind of noise-blocking machine with soothing sounds can also help. One patient of mine has lights with a motion sensor in her backyard. Any time a neighborhood cat or her own dog is out there prowling around in the middle of the night, the lights flick on, often awakening her. This is the kind of situation in which a mask can help. And speaking of animals, just say no to dogs and cats sleeping on your bed. Not only can their propensity to hog space and move around at their leisure be disturbing, but they can also leave behind hair and dander that stir up allergies and asthma. Love your pet, but get him his own bed. The importance of darkness, quiet, and the absence of movement in your bedroom can't be overstated.

7. Seek a Solution for Snoring

Snoring can be a sign of sleep apnea, which I discuss on page 192, as well as physiological irregularities (such as large tonsils) that cause breathing to vibrate the soft palate in the back of the mouth. It's always wise to have your doctor evaluate you to determine the underlying cause of your snoring, even if it's not disturbing your sleep. Some people snore loudly and don't wake themselves up (although their bed partners aren't always so fortunate).

If your snoring isn't associated with a health problem such as obstructive sleep apnea and you're just seeking ways to lessen your bed partner's sleep disruption, there are a few remedies you can try. One is to nix alcohol at night, which can exacerbate snoring. Another is to lose weight if needed: Overweight people tend to be more susceptible to snoring (and sleep apnea). You might also try sleeping on your stomach or side (sleeping on your stomach does make your face more prone to wrinkles, but it can also decrease snoring). If you can't seem to stay off your back, try sleeping in a T-shirt with a tennis ball sewn into a pocket between your shoulder blades. Nasal strips have also been shown to help diminish snoring by increasing airflow through the nostrils. For stubborn cases, there are surgical options. Some ear, nose, and throat specialists even offer "snoreplasty," a procedure that involves injecting a stiffening agent into the soft palate.

8. Arm Yourself with a Good Mattress and Pillow

Comfort is key to a good night's sleep. Pillows are a personal preference — some people like hard, flat ones; others like them soft and fluffy — but make sure that you buy one that won't aggravate allergies or asthma if you have either. Look for pillows without feathers or those billed as "hypoallergenic." You can also purchase pillow casings that block out dust mites, which can lead to allergy or asthma reactions, too. If you have arthritis in your neck, check out cervical pillows, specially made curved supports for the neck.

Like pillows, mattresses too are a personal preference. However, whatever kind you choose, be certain that it allows your head and spine to be aligned when you lie down (your hips shouldn't sink). Consider a memory foam mattress. It is designed to mold to the curves of your body. This can put less stress on your bones and muscles and decrease orthopedic-related aches and pains that develop with age. An added benefit to memory foam is that you won't disrupt your bed partner's sleep as you change positions through the night.

When you shop for a mattress, test it out by lying down in your typical

Help! It's Three A.M. and I Can't Sleep

"I wake up at three in the morning. I lie in bed and can't get back to sleep." I hear that complaint in my office just about every day, especially among patients over the ages of forty and fifty who are just beginning to feel the effects of the age-related downturn in stage 3 sleep. So what is to be done?

Don't just lie in bed looking at the clock—in fact, don't look at the clock at all. That will only make you anxious ("I have to get up in three hours!"), and anxiety is the enemy of sleep because it leads to the production of arousing chemicals in the body. Worrying about not being able to sleep makes it a self-fulfilling prophecy. Get out of bed—you don't want your bed to become a place you associate with sleeplessness. Sit quietly in another room with a dim light, open up a magazine or book (preferably something a little boring), and when you begin to feel sleepy, turn off the light and go back to bed. If it happens again, repeat.

There are all kinds of reasons you may wake up in the middle of the night or very early in the morning, including disturbing sounds or lights, having to go to the bathroom, hot flashes, pain from arthritis or other conditions. Wakefulness is also a common symptom of depression, so if you're constantly battling insomnia, think about what other symptoms you might have. Prolonged bouts of sadness, frequent crying, feelings of worthlessness, and finding that you don't enjoy life are all signs of depression (and the risk of depression, we know, increases with age). Seek help if you have any of these symptoms, and seek help immediately if you're having thoughts of harming yourself.

sleep position, then before you buy make sure the mattress has a thirty-day warranty. That way if it turns out to be not so comfortable after all, you can exchange it for another.

9. Try a Sleep Aid

Sleeping pills can be very helpful as a short-term treatment for insomnia. Sometimes an emotional event—say you've lost a spouse or are getting married—can trigger acute insomnia; once you've gotten over the worst part of grieving or the excitement of a wedding, the bad sleeping habits you developed may remain and lead to a chronic problem with insomnia. Many modern sleeping pills are effective and nonaddictive, and they can be just the thing to get your sleep back on track if you're going through a rough patch.

Sleeping pills, though, shouldn't be the first thing you try when you're having chronic trouble sleeping—make sure you have all the other sleep hygiene habits in place first. Another option is to consider several thirty-minute sessions of cognitive behavioral therapy (CBT). Psychiatrists, psychologists, and other trained counselors often use CBT to treat insomnia related to anxiety and distorted thinking (i.e., you tend to blow small problems out of proportion). It can be very helpful and may end your need for sleeping pills altogether.

If sleeping pills remain a consideration, it's worth consulting your doctor about benzodiazepine-like hypnotics (such as Ambien, Sonata, and Lunesta) and benzodiazepines (such as Restoril, Ativan, and Klonopin). Benzodiazepines have multiple uses—they're also prescribed as muscle relaxants and anti-anxiety drugs—and they can be especially helpful if besides insomnia you have restless legs syndrome or another disorder called periodic limb movements, in which your legs move rhythmically at night. They're a good choice if you also suffer from anxiety, but shouldn't be used if you have sleep apnea (they can suppress respiration).

While both types of drugs can cause a dependency, benzodiazepine-like hypnotics cause fewer withdrawal symptoms. Bear in mind that both types of drugs can have side effects such as residual drowsiness during the day, a decrease in hand-eye coordination, and sleepwalking (and even sleep eating, cooking, and driving). You might also talk to your doctor about using other non-sleeping-pill medications to help you sleep. Antidepressants, other types of muscle relaxants, and antihistamines can all be useful for insomnia (although some antidepressants can have the opposite effect).

Melatonin supplements work for some people, too. Melatonin is a hormone naturally secreted by the body that plays a role in establishing the sleep-wake cycle and that declines with age. Whereas light tells the body to wake up, melatonin tells the body to go to sleep. If you're going to try melatonin supplements, do so with caution, because melatonin can disturb your circadian rhythm more than you'd like. Start with a low dose (1.5 mg), then slowly increase the dosage if you find you need more. Don't exceed 6 mg a day, and never take it if you're pregnant or have a serious medical condition.

Valerian is another alternative sleep aid you might talk to your doctor about. It seems to have Valium-like effects in most people, but be aware that some find it stimulating. Be cautious; start with a dose lower than that recommended on the label (it comes in extract, tablet, and capsule form), and see how it goes before increasing your dosage.

10. Minimize Jet Lag

If you cross time zones, you can end up with a temporary circadian rhythm disorder (jet lag). What happens is that your body stays in the time zone you just left even though there are cues around you (such as daylight or darkness) indicating that you're now on a different schedule. As a result, you can end up overly sleepy or unable to sleep. You may even have gastrointestinal problems. To reduce jet lag when you're flying east, once you reach your destination, seek exposure to light in the morning; this will help your circadian rhythm catch up. If you're flying west, seek exposure to light (even artificial light) in the evening. Using a sleep aid to make it easier to get some shut-eye while you're flying or to deal with the time change once you've arrived can also be helpful.

You can further help yourself push past jet lag by making sure your accommodations are conducive to a good night's sleep. Call in advance to ask for a hotel room that's quiet — no elevators, workout rooms, or ice machines next door, no windows overlooking the pool or flashing neon signs. In a city, ask to be on a high floor (farther away from traffic) and in a room that doesn't face a busy street. Then, as much as possible, treat your hotel room as you do your own bedroom. Go through the same before-bed rituals you do at home.

11. Play Catch Up

As I said earlier, consistency is key in overcoming sleep obstacles. But on occasions when it's impossible to maintain your regular habits, you can still catch up on sleep. This is known as paying your sleep debt. Sleeping longer on weekends or napping (see page 200) will let you make up for some of the hours you've lost; however, be aware that either can throw you off schedule again. Work on getting back into your regular routine and try to avoid the need to play catch up very often.

———————

Remember, a good night's sleep is something you can't afford to take for granted. Deep, refreshing sleep is vital to your health and sense of well-being. It's integral to fighting the effects of aging, including the risk of diseases that are more likely to crop up as you get older. Inadequate sleep can definitely shorten your life.

If you're not motivated by the fear of a life-threatening disease, at least consider how much better you feel when you're well rested. Sleep improves the quality of your life in every way. The brightness and resiliency of your skin. Your memory and ability to concentrate. Your mood. Your level of get-up-and-go. How well you eat. How much energy you have for exercise.

Use the suggestions in this chapter to help you develop good habits before difficulties arise. Just like all the other pillars of anti-aging in this book, effective sleep habits require discipline and commitment. You need to purposefully manage your day and evening, and you may even have to give up certain cherished rituals to get the results you need. But give yourself the gift of a good night's sleep and you're sure to improve your health and the overall quality of your life.

CHAPTER 6

The Art of Aging Gracefully

None are so old as those who have outlived enthusiasm.

—Henry David Thoreau

THE PHRASE "AGING GRACEFULLY" gets tossed around a lot. But what does aging gracefully really mean? Images from the big screen may leap to mind. There are many actors and actresses — Cary Grant, Paul Newman, Katharine Hepburn, Sophia Loren, Raquel Welch, Meryl Streep, Diane Keaton, Sidney Poitier, Sean Connery, to name a few — whose looks and demeanor remained, and remain, vibrant with age. But what strikes me most about people who have transcended their chronological age is that they exude a certain joie de vivre — joy of living. Aging gracefully to me means continuing to be enthusiastic about life and all that it has to offer. The most compelling reason to hang on to your health, maintain strength and energy, and, yes, even look your best, is that it helps you stay positive and be happy, active, excited, and in love with life.

Youth has many blessings, so of course we try to stay young. But age has its rewards, too, and they are often overlooked or, at best, viewed as sort of a consolation prize. Yet the experience, knowledge, and judgment you gain as you grow older are wonderful gifts. And I'm not just talking about the proverbial wisdom of the wizened ninety-year-old. These are things that you begin to lay claim to as you move into your forties, fifties, and beyond. When you're younger, a lot of your energy goes into defining yourself. You're learning about yourself and what you want from life. In the later stages of life, you will have hopefully figured out who you are, and that allows you to focus your energy on the things that make you feel happy and satisfied.

It's easy to lament the things we did or didn't do in our earlier years, and even to still feel stuck — maybe you never lost the weight you wanted to, never attained the professional heights you desired, are still in a toxic relationship, or have never found the right significant other. But it's never too late to change your life: to improve your health, break with someone who is making you unhappy, or continue to meet new people. You can even change your career path, or perhaps go back to school to expand your interests and knowledge. Part of aging gracefully is zeroing in on not only what is important to you, but who is truly important to you, and letting the rest fall by the wayside. Nurturing meaningful relationships is particularly critical: those relationships can help you live longer — and certainly better.

THE BENEFIT OF FRIENDS

Certainly, one of the most significant relationships, if not the most significant relationship, you can have is the relationship with yourself. That means, among other things, to be aware of your own thoughts and feelings and to be giving to (and forgiving of) yourself. Having a good relationship with yourself not only makes you a psychologically healthier person, but helps open the door to good relationships with other people as well. And that's essential: The love, friendship, and companionship of others is integral to aging gracefully. It's well known that isolation or perceived loneliness is associated with conditions that age the body and put it at greater risk of age-related diseases. Loneliness, for instance, has been found to raise blood pressure, affect sleep quality, and increase the production of the stress hormone cortisol. On the other hand, friendship (even more than family relationships) has been associated with decreases in depression, increases in self-esteem, and better coping with stress.

Data from the Australian Longitudinal Study of Aging has shown that people age seventy and older who have an active social life live 22 percent

Make Your Brain More Age-Resistant

Taking care of your mental well-being by reducing stress, finding sources of happiness in everyday life, and adjusting your perceptions of aging are all important ways to keep your brain healthy. Many of the things you do for overall health—exercising, eating well, getting adequate sleep—can help, too. But there are practical strategies that can protect your brain from decline. Here are some that have been shown to help.

Learn something new. There's been some suggestion that mentally challenging or stimulating activities such as puzzles keep the brain sharp. Sorry, crossword fans. "There's no evidence that people who do crossword puzzles regularly have better cognitive function," says Denise Park, PhD, director of the Center for Vital Longevity in Dallas. "It may be that this type of activity doesn't involve creating new knowledge—you're passively entering in definitions of words you already know." However, when you learn something completely new, you can create new pathways or neural circuits in the brain—almost like scaffolding around the brain. What might work? Learning a new language, a new instrument, a new computer program—check out your local adult education campus to see all the possibilities.

Be safe. Anything that puts strain or stress on your head can, over time, damage your brain. This includes the obvious dangers—skiing or hiking without a helmet or driving without a seatbelt, for instance—as well as the more unexpected ones, for example, heading a soccer ball. "It's important to be conscious of activities that may seem to have nothing to do with the brain but can cause damage that aggregates over a lifetime. Keep in mind that even minimal blows to the head can cause trouble," says Park.

Be active. I'll repeat what I said in more detail in chapter 2 (see page 32): People who exercise have better blood flow to the brain, they produce substances that foster the growth of new brain cells, and they're at a lower risk for Alzheimer's.

Get your fill of omega-3 fats. Your brain is surrounded by a flexible, fluid membrane that's made up of omega-3 fatty acids. When you don't get enough of these healthy fats from your diet, your body uses omega-6 fats, which are less pliable and slow reactions in the brain. For more on omega-3s, see page 107.

longer than those with a less active social life. And in 2008, researchers at Harvard's School of Public Health found that socially active seniors had a slower rate of memory decline than their more isolated peers.

These studies looked at people who were elderly, but they point out the importance of cultivating relationships and staying socially active right *now*. Every chapter in this book has been devoted not only to helping you shave years off your present physiological age but to helping you develop healthy habits that will hold you in good stead in the future. Tending to your relationships is part of that and just as important as exercising and eating right.

Take this as your cue to continue widening your circle of friends as the years go by. Anything that keeps you socially active now — joining a book club or walking group, taking classes at a local high school or community center, meeting up regularly with friends or colleagues — will pay off later. Personally, I've seen the value of having a diverse group of friends, some younger than I am and some older than I am. As my parents have gotten older, I've watched as many of their friends have passed away. So from a practical standpoint, having friends from different generations ensures you'll have company and support well into your later years. But there's another perk. In a way, youthfulness is contagious. When you bond with people younger than yourself, they keep you up to date on changes taking place in the world — new technology, say, or the latest in art, or even changes in the English language. I think a reluctance to try new things contributes to more rapid aging. When you have younger friends, it broadens your horizons. You don't just look back — you look forward, and that helps to keep you interested in life.

ATTITUDE AND AGING

Though age can help you become more certain about your character, individuality, spirituality — your overall place and purpose in this world — it can also make you feel out of the mainstream. So much in our culture celebrates and idealizes youth while often reducing older people to a punch line, sometimes even infantilizing those in their later years. It's so important to resist the stereotypes that equate aging with a loss of relevance.

One person who has written eloquently about the role of self-perception in aging is Sherwin B. Nuland, MD, a surgeon and author. "If there is a single factor that is the foundation stone for all successful aging, a factor that allows every other element, encourages every other element, and nurtures every other element, that factor must surely be a healthy self-image," Dr. Nuland wrote in *The Art of Aging*. "We need to approve of ourselves, to take pride in what we have become, to feel a vibrancy in our moral sense — we must, quite simply, be happy with what we are."

Thinking that you're "past your prime" or that you're edging toward being "over the hill" even as you're just moving out of your forties has the potential to become a self-fulfilling prophecy. Evidence suggests that how you view aging significantly affects your ability to stay healthy, active, and on the ball. It may even affect how long you live.

A great example of how attitude influences actuality is a well-known experiment called the Counterclockwise Study. In 1979, the psychologist Ellen Langer and her students at Harvard University devised a study that involved having frail, elderly men spend a week living in a monastery outfitted to look as though it were still the year 1959. The furnishings and everything the men experienced, from the television programs they watched and the music they heard to the newspapers they read and daily discussions they had fit into a twenty-year time warp.

The men were split into two groups, and the first group was instructed not just to *act* like it was 1959, but as much as possible to *be* who they were in 1959. To set the stage, they were asked to write a biography of themselves in the present tense as if it were twenty years earlier. A week later, the second group of participants took their turn in the retro environment, but instead of living as if it were 1959, they were told to live in the present and simply reminisce about the past. They also wrote bios about who they were in 1959, but in the past tense. Despite being extremely dependent on relatives prior to the study, at the study's end, both sets of seniors were able to function independently. Having to live on their own, being treated with respect and engaging in lively discussions had had an obvious effect on them. Both groups also improved their hearing and memory after the week's retreat. But the group who lived as if they were twenty years younger reaped even more benefits: They had more joint flexibility, scored better on intelligence tests, and had better posture and gait. By many measures, they actually got younger. "It is not primarily our physical selves that limit us but rather our mindset about our physical limits," concluded Langer.

Since Langer weighed in with the Counterclockwise Study, other researchers have shown that attitude can have considerable power over how well someone ages. For instance, Thomas Hess, PhD, a professor in the graduate program on Lifespan Developmental Psychology in the Department of Psychology at North Carolina State University, and his team had two groups of older folks read bogus newspaper articles about aging and memory to see if it had any influence on their own memories. One group read about a scientific paper that found people have a lot of control over memory as they age, while the other group read an article stating that memory declines as you get older and there's not much you can do about it. After completing their reading, both groups were given a list of thirty words to study for two minutes, then were asked to recall as many words as they could. The group that read the positive article recalled 10 to 15 percent more words than the group who read the negative article. If this study is any indication, believing that it's possible to retain brain power as you age can make it a reality—but believing the opposite can cause your mental aptitude to diminish. "What's more, one thing that's emerging is how important it is to maintain an engaged lifestyle and exercise cognitive skills," says Dr. Hess. "If you fall prey to negative stereotypes, you may remove yourself from situations that require these skills, and this would exacerbate any normal cognitive changes you'd see."

There's one more study I want to tell you about because it illustrates how important it is not to buy in to the notion that it's all downhill once you're past middle age. Recently, Becca Levy, PhD, an associate professor of epidemiology and psychology at Yale University, followed up on some data collected back in the 1970s by a gerontologist in Oxford, Ohio. The gerontologist surveyed more than one thousand people ages fifty and older in the town and had them answer a variety of questions regarding their health, work, and lifestyle. One of the questions included in the survey was what the townspeople thought of aging. Many years later, Levy and her team looked at their answers to this question, then tracked down mortality information about the people to see if there was any correlation between attitude and life span. What they found was that people who believed that aging was a positive experience tended to live seven and a half years longer. This suggests that there really is a connection between attitude and longevity.

THE HAPPINESS FACTOR

If I had to boil down all of the sociopsychological factors that help you age gracefully into one word, that word would be *happiness*. It's happiness — that joie de vivre I mentioned earlier — that makes all the difference.

The good news is that many people actually *are* happier as they get older. When researchers at the Centers for Disease Control and Prevention (CDC) surveyed different age groups about happiness, they found that people in their early twenties reported feeling sad on an average of 3.4 days per month, while people aged sixty-five to seventy-four felt sad 2.3 days. There are probably a lot of reasons for the difference. When you're older you're generally freed from child rearing and the stress of building and maintaining a career. You also tend to have more coping skills at your disposal — you've been through stressful experiences before and know how to handle them. Experience also teaches you that life is cyclical. Things may get bad, but they usually get better again. When you're young and haven't lived through so many ups and downs, you're not as likely to see the sun on the horizon.

We instinctively know that happiness is healthier for us, but there is also hard evidence that it can slow the effects of aging. For instance, happiness can help strengthen your immune system. Researchers at Rush University Medical Center in Chicago, now conducting one of the largest ongoing studies on Alzheimer's and aging, have found that people who reported having a greater sense of purpose and direction in life (to me that's longhand for happiness) also have a lower risk for Alzheimer's disease and cognitive deterioration. Happy people are also at a much lower risk of premature death, according to a study published in the *Journal of Health Psychology.* "I think we underestimate the importance of being happy. There's not a lot of research on happiness and brain functioning right now, but I expect we'll soon learn that there are real relationships between high life satisfaction and brain health," says Denise Park.

One thing is for sure: People who suffer from depression experience an impairment in concentration and attention — it's as if their brain is aging. "In fact, depression can sometimes first appear as a memory problem, like a pseudo dementia," says Cynthia Green, PhD, a brain health expert and assistant clinical professor of psychiatry at Mount Sinai School of Medicine in New York City. And depression also seems to be connected to real dementia. Some research shows that women who are depressed are more likely to suffer dementia later in life.

While it's good news that the CDC survey found that older people have a higher rate of happy days, happiness is not something you want to save for your senior years. It's important to pursue it now. Aside from the fact that it simply feels better to be happy, it's going to help you retain your health and continue to function at a high level. If you don't feel happy, examining your life to discover why is just as important an anti-aging strategy as anything else we've recommended in this book. You may find that you need to make big changes in your life (changes, for instance, in a relationship or your job), but you may also find that you simply need to take more time to experience joy, to add more elements of surprise and adventure to your life, or to live more purposefully or compassionately. There are a lot of keys to happiness; determine the key to yours.

ACTIVELY PARTICIPATING IN LIFE

Recently, I've read about a couple of teachers who are still in the classroom even though they are in their nineties. To me this is another strategy for aging well: continuing to be an active participant in life. This doesn't necessarily mean you have to keep working until you're in your nineties; it simply means being engaged with the world. Taking yourself off autopilot. Many people go through the day somewhat unaware of what's going on around them. They may commute to work hardly noticing the other cars or the people riding next to them on the bus or train. They might sit in a meeting without ever really paying attention to who's around them or what they're wearing. Think about it: What color is the carpet in your office? Who lives on the corner of your street? Who is your congressional representative? These things might seem inconsequential, but if you're unaware of them, it shows just how passive and disconnected you can become.

And yet living a more engaged life can really pay off when it comes to longevity and vitality. "If people are engaged in life, they're more likely to maintain their cognitive skills," explains Thomas Hess. "Studies funded by the National Institute on Aging show that what people do in midlife — their jobs, their leisure activities — has a pretty strong effect on cognitive changes later on." Anything that calls for you to use your brain and make decisions can help you maintain your cognitive abilities.

There's a deep connection between what I've been talking about in this chapter — staying positive, not giving in to negative stereotypes about aging, seeking happiness and companionship — and everything else in this book. When you are physically fit, eating and sleeping well, and looking your best, you simply function at a higher level and for that reason you feel good. That in turn makes you ten thousand times more likely to graciously accept growing older, to even welcome it in many ways.

There's no question that staving off the effects of aging takes work and possibly changing some ingrained habits. The truth is, many people passively let physical and psychological decline invade their lives as they grow older. When you put in the time and energy to stay strong, healthy, and enthusiastic, it can transform you in profound physical *and* emotional ways. When your body is strong and you feel your best, you become more engaged in the world and appreciative of the people around you. Life simply seems more beautiful.

One thing many people don't realize when they're younger — but which becomes crystal clear with age — is that life is incredibly precious. Every moment counts. You have it within you to live each of those moments to the fullest. If you make the decision to keep your body and mind in the best possible shape, it's going to help ensure that your time on this earth is not only long but, most important, well lived.

PART II

THE 20 YEARS YOUNGER LIFESTYLE

CHAPTER 7

Meal Plans and Recipes

MUCH OF WHAT RESEARCH HAS TOLD US about what helps stave off the aging process is incorporated into the following two-week eating plan. Think of it as your introduction to an easy, effective, and terrific-tasting way to turn back the clock. After the two weeks are over, you can repeat the meal plans again, or simply use them as a template to create your own healthy plan. If you choose to do the latter, use the guidelines on page 89 and below as well as the list of superfoods in chapter 3 to help you continue eating for longevity and optimal energy.

Most of the meals on the plan take between three and twenty minutes to prepare, and all the ingredients are easily found in your local supermarket. Here's how it works.

- Pick a daily calorie level: 1,500, 1,700, 2,000, or 2,500. For help figuring out the right calorie level, turn to page 91.

- You can swap one meal for another as long as they're equivalent, e.g. the breakfast in Day 1 for the breakfast in Day 7. Same goes for the other meals, snacks, and treats. A day's plan might include Day 1's breakfast, Day 5's lunch, Day 6's dinner, a snack from Day 11, and a treat from Day 14. This way, you keep creating new meal plans, allowing you to stretch out these menus for months.

- Check my website 20YearsYounger.com for more support, recipes, and meal ideas.

- It's okay to substitute foods that are similar for one another. For instance, you can have almonds in place of walnuts, chicken for lamb, green peppers for broccoli. This will give your diet more variety.

- Soy milk, nonfat (skim) milk and 1% milk are interchangeable — so if there's soy milk in a meal and you'd rather have nonfat or 1% milk, go ahead and make the swap.

- If you need more salt, add it sparingly to the food on your plate, not to the entire dish. This will give you saltiness without as much sodium. No matter how you swap and combine meals, this plan is designed to max out at 2,300 mg sodium. Remember, for each ⅛ teaspoon of salt you add, you're adding 290 mg more sodium. Take out a measuring spoon, measure out ⅛ teaspoon and put it in your hand so you know what that amount looks like. Then get rid of half of it. What's left is the amount you should add to your meal — even less if possible.

- If you want to design your own meals, use the calorie guide in the chart below. Each day, make sure to have several servings of fruits or vegetables, a serving or two of whole grains, and two servings of nonfat or 1% milk or soy milk (or three if you're on 2,500 calories/day). Stick to lean sources of protein and healthy fats as well.

Calories Per Day	Calories Per Meal/Snack/Treat					
	Breakfast	Lunch	Dinner	Snack 1	Snack 2	Treat
1,500	400	425	525	150	None	None
1,700	440	430	525	155	None	150
2,000	440	565	645	150	None	200
2,500	440	660	750	150	250	250

- If you find through trial and error that your ideal daily calorie level is one we don't offer (for instance 1,800 calories or 3,000 calories), follow the closest *lower* calorie level and *add* foods from the list below. Here's an example of how to make the appropriate adjustments. If you think you need 1,800 calories per day, follow the 1,700 calories/day plan and add 100 more calories through foods from the list. If you need 3,000 calories per day, make the 2,500 calories/day your base and bolster it with 500 more daily calories. One easy way to do this is to simply double up on the two snacks offered on the plan — one is 150 calories, the other 250, so that gives you 400 extra calories — then add another 100 calories from the list below.

Healthful Ways to Bulk Up on Calories

FRUIT

(*60 calories per serving*)

A serving is...

Apple — 1 medium

Apricots — 4 fresh or 8 dried halves

Banana ½

Berries (blackberries, blueberries, strawberries, raspberries) — 1 cup

Cantaloupe — 1 cup chopped

Cherries — 14

Dates — 3

Figs — 2 medium fresh or 1½ dried

Fruit salad — 1 cup chopped

Grapefruit — ½

Grapes — ½ cup

Kiwi — 1½

Orange — 1 small

Mango — ½ or ½ cup slices

Peach — 1 medium

Pear — 1 small

Pineapple — ¾ cup cubes

VEGETABLES

(*25 calories per serving*)

A serving is…

Asparagus — 8 spears

Bean sprouts — ¾ cup

Beets — ½ cup cooked

Broccoli — 1 cup raw or ½ cup cooked

Cabbage — 1½ cups raw shredded or ¾ cup cooked

Carrot — 1 medium or ½ cup chopped

Cauliflower — 1 cup raw or cooked

Celery — 4 medium stalks

Cucumber — 1½ cups sliced

Eggplant — 1 cup cooked

Greens (such as collard, kale, spinach, turnip greens) — ½ cup cooked

Lettuce (such as arugula, mixed greens, romaine) — 3 cups

String beans — ½ cup cooked

Tomato — 1 medium, ¾ cup chopped or 1 cup cherry tomatoes

Tomato sauce (plain) — ⅓ cup

WHOLE GRAINS/STARCHY VEGETABLES

(*80 calories per serving*)

A serving is…

Bagel, whole wheat — ¼ of a large bagel or ½ a medium

Beans (legumes, such as black beans, pinto beans, white beans, garbanzos, lentils) — ⅓ cup cooked or canned

Bread, 100% whole grain — 1 slice with at least 2 grams fiber

Bulgur wheat — ½ cup cooked

Cereal, flaky type — about ¾ cup (at least 4 grams fiber per 100 calories)

Corn — ½ cup or 5-inch ear

Couscous, whole wheat (such as Fantastic Foods or Casbah) — ½ cup cooked

Crispbread, whole grain — 80 calories' worth and no more than 2 grams fat

English muffin, whole wheat — ½

Grits — ½ cup cooked

Muesli — ¼ cup

Muffin, bran or whole grain — ¼ large muffin, or ½ of a 2.75×2-inch-diameter muffin

Oatmeal, plain (or other unsweetened whole-grain hot cereal) — ½ cup cooked

Pancake, whole grain — 2 pancakes with a 4-inch diameter

Pasta, whole grain — ½ cup cooked

Peas — ¾ cup

Pita bread, whole wheat — ½ of a 6-inch round

Polenta — ⅓ cup cooked

Popcorn — 3 cups (air popped or no more than 3 grams fat)

Potato or sweet potato — ½ medium, or heaping ½ cup cooked with no fat added

Roll, whole wheat — 1 small (1 ounce) or ½ of a 65-gram (2.3 ounces) hamburger roll

Rice, brown or wild — ⅓ cup cooked

Tortilla — 1 tortilla (7 inches)

Waffles, whole grain — one small frozen waffle or four ½-inch squares

LEAN PROTEIN

(about 60 calories per serving)

A serving is…

Beef, lean (such as sirloin, tenderloin, and 95 percent lean ground) — 1 ounce cooked

Cheese, reduced-fat hard (such as reduced-fat cheddar, jack, or Swiss) — 1 ounce (no more than 3 grams of saturated fat per ounce)

Chicken, skinless — 1½ ounces or ¼ cup diced broiled, or 1 ounce or 3 tablespoons diced stewed

Egg — 1 large

Eggs, liquid (such as Better'n Eggs) — ½ cup

Fish, white-fleshed (such as grouper, flounder, or snapper) — 2 ounces cooked

Fish, oily (such as salmon, trout, or bluefish) — 1 ounce cooked

Peanut butter (such as Smart Balance) — 1 tablespoon (also counts as 1 fat serving)

Pork tenderloin — 1 ounce

Salmon, canned, packed in water, drained — 2 ounces

Seitan (wheat protein) — 2 ounces

Tempeh (fermented soy) — 1¼ ounces

Tofu — 2 to 4 ounces (check label as calories vary)

Tuna, canned, light, packed in water, drained — 2 ounces

Vegetable burger, soy based — ½ patty (check label as products differ; ideally, the entire burger should have at least 12 grams of protein and no more than 9 grams of carbohydrate, which you must count toward your grain/starchy vegetable servings)

HEALTHY FATS

(45 calories per serving)

A serving is...

Avocado — ⅛ of a whole avocado

Margarine — 1 teaspoon (with no partially hydrogenated oil, such as Bestlife buttery spread)

Margarine, light — 1 tablespoon (with no partially hydrogenated oil)

Mayonnaise, reduced fat — 1 tablespoon

Nuts, any kind — 1 tablespoon

Nut butter — 1½ teaspoons

Oil (such as olive oil or canola oil) — 1 teaspoon

Ricotta cheese — 1½ tablespoons

Ricotta cheese, part skim — 2 tablespoons

Salad dressing — 2 teaspoons to 1 tablespoon

Salad dressing, reduced fat — 1 to 2 tablespoons (check label for calorie counts)

MENUS

Day 1

Breakfast

1,700, 2,000, AND 2,500 CALORIES/DAY:

- *Acai Almond Butter Smoothie:* In a blender, combine until smooth 1 package (100 grams) frozen acai, ½ cup frozen unsweetened raspberries, 1 tablespoon almond butter, 2 teaspoons honey, 1 cup skim milk, and 1 tablespoon ground flaxseed.

- Sprinkle ¼ cup whole grain cereal such as Kashi Good Friends on top of smoothie.

1,500 CALORIES/DAY: Omit the cereal.

Lunch

1,500 AND 1,700 CALORIES/DAY:

- *Sardine Salad:* 3 cups shredded romaine lettuce, 2 ounces sardines packed in olive oil and drained, tossed with 2 teaspoons lemon juice, 1 tablespoon finely chopped red onion, and 2 tablespoons finely chopped Italian parsley.

- A 1-ounce whole wheat roll (about 73 calories), torn and dipped in 2 teaspoons olive oil.

- Serve with ¾ cup grapes and 2 medium fresh or dried figs.

2,000 CALORIES/DAY: Serve Sardine Salad with 1½ ounce whole wheat roll (about 109 calories), torn and dipped in 1 tablespoon olive oil. Serve with 1½ cup grapes and 3 medium fresh or dried figs.

2,500 CALORIES/DAY: Serve Sardine Salad with 1½ ounce whole wheat roll (about 109 calories), torn and dipped in 1 tablespoon olive oil. Serve with 1½ cup grapes, 3 medium fresh or dried figs, and 1½ tablespoons chopped pecans.

Dinner

1,500 AND 1,700 CALORIES/DAY:

- 1 serving Baked Eggplant and Ground Turkey (page 259).

- ½ cup cooked cracked wheat (bulgur) with 2 teaspoons olive oil, a pinch of salt, black pepper to taste, and 1 tablespoon finely chopped fresh basil.

- 2 cups baby spinach dressed with 1 teaspoon olive oil, ½ teaspoon balsamic vinegar, and black pepper to taste.

- ¾ cup chopped cantaloupe.

2,000 CALORIES/DAY: 1 serving Baked Eggplant and Ground Turkey with ½ cup cooked cracked wheat (bulgur) tossed with 1 tablespoon olive oil, a pinch of salt, black pepper to taste, and 1 tablespoon finely chopped fresh basil. Serve with spinach salad and cantaloupe as noted above.

2,500 CALORIES/DAY: 1 serving Baked Eggplant and Ground Turkey with ¾ cup cooked cracked wheat (bulgur) with 1 tablespoon olive oil, a pinch of salt, black pepper to taste, and 1 tablespoon finely chopped fresh basil. Serve with spinach salad and cantaloupe as noted above.

Snack

ALL CALORIE LEVELS:

- *Fresh Mint Tea:* 2 tablespoons fresh mint steeped in 1¼ cups hot soy milk and then strained (can also be chilled for iced tea). Sweeten with 1 teaspoon honey.

2,500 CALORIES/DAY EXTRA SNACK: 1 medium apple sliced and spread with 2 tablespoons sunflower seed butter.

Treat

1,500 CALORIES/DAY: Omit the treat.

1,700 CALORIES/DAY:

- *Graham Cracker with Banana and Walnuts:* Top 1 graham cracker (2 squares) with ½ sliced banana and 1 tablespoon chopped walnuts.

2,000 CALORIES/DAY: Top 2 graham crackers with ½ sliced banana and 2 teaspoons chopped walnuts.

2,500 CALORIES/DAY: Top 2 graham crackers with ½ sliced banana and 1 tablespoon plus 2 teaspoons chopped walnuts.

Day 2

Breakfast

1,500 CALORIES/DAY:

- 1 serving Muesli (page 255) served with 1 cup skim milk and topped with ½ cup fresh blackberries.

1,700, 2,000, AND 2,500 CALORIES/DAY:

- 1 serving Muesli served with 1 cup skim milk and topped with ½ cup fresh blackberries and 1½ tablespoons chopped almonds.

Lunch

1,500 AND 1,700 CALORIES/DAY:

- Chicken, Grapefruit, and Arugula Salad: Combine 2 ounces dark meat or 3 ounces light meat rotisserie chicken, bones and skin removed, and cut into strips, 3 cups arugula, sections from 1 grapefruit, skin and pith removed, 1½ teaspoons olive oil, 1 teaspoon cider vinegar, and black pepper to taste.

- 2 Wasa multigrain crispbreads topped with 1 teaspoon Bestlife spread.

2,000 CALORIES/DAY: Make salad as above but with 2.75 ounces dark meat or 4 ounces of light meat rotisserie chicken and topped with 1 tablespoon cashew halves. Serve with 2 Wasa multigrain crispbreads spread with 1 teaspoon Bestlife spread.

2,500 CALORIES/DAY: Make salad as above but with 2.75 ounces dark meat or 4 ounces light meat rotisserie chicken and topped with 2 tablespoons cashew halves and 2½ tablespoons golden raisins. Serve with 2 Wasa multigrain crispbreads prepared as above.

Dinner

1,500 AND 1,700 CALORIES/DAY:

- 1 serving Poached Trout with Tomato and Basil (page 262).

- Spicy Farro or Barley with Mint and Parsley: Dress 1 cup grain cooked according to package directions with 2 teaspoons olive oil, ¼ cup cooked shiitake mushrooms, a large pinch of cayenne pepper, a pinch of salt, 2 tablespoons finely chopped fresh mint, and 2 tablespoons finely chopped curly parsley.

- 1 cup fresh sliced strawberries.

2,000 CALORIES/DAY: 1 serving Poached Trout with Tomato and Basil with 1½ cups cooked farro or barley tossed with 2½ teaspoons olive oil, ¼ cup cooked shiitake mushrooms, a large pinch of cayenne pepper, a pinch of salt, 3 tablespoons finely chopped fresh mint, and 3 tablespoons finely chopped curly parsley. Serve with 1 cup fresh sliced strawberries.

2,500 CALORIES/DAY: 1 serving Poached Trout with Tomato and Basil with 1¾ cups cooked farro or barley tossed with 1 tablespoon olive oil, ¼ cup cooked shiitake mushrooms, a large pinch of cayenne pepper, a pinch of salt, 3 tablespoons finely chopped fresh mint, and 3 tablespoons finely chopped curly parsley. Serve with 1½ cups fresh sliced strawberries.

Snack

ALL CALORIE LEVELS:

- Pomegranate Freeze: In a blender, blend until smooth (about 30 seconds) ¼ cup frozen 100% pomegranate juice (freeze in ice cube tray or paper cup) and 1¼ cups plain soy milk.

2,500 CALORIES/DAY EXTRA SNACK: 1 small 4-inch whole wheat pita bread spread with 1 tablespoon plus 2 teaspoons no-salt-added almond butter.

Treat

1,500 CALORIES/DAY: Omit the treat.

1,700 CALORIES/DAY:

- 1 serving Zucchini Olive Oil Cake (page 270).

2,000 CALORIES/DAY: 1 serving Zucchini Olive Oil Cake with ¼ cup plus 2 tablespoons unsweetened applesauce.

2,500 CALORIES/DAY: 1 serving Zucchini Olive Oil Cake with 1 cup unsweetened applesauce.

Day 3

Breakfast

1,500 CALORIES/DAY:

- ¾ cup shredded wheat topped with 1 tablespoon ground flaxseed, 1½ tablespoons chopped walnuts, ¾ cup sliced strawberries, and 1 cup plain soy milk.

1,700, 2,000, AND 2,500 CALORIES/DAY: 1 cup shredded wheat topped with 1 tablespoon ground flaxseed, 2 tablespoons chopped walnuts, ¾ cup sliced strawberries, and 1 cup plain soy milk.

Lunch

1,500 AND 1,700 CALORIES/DAY:

- Edamame Dip: 1 cup cooked shelled edamame pureed in a food processor with 2 teaspoons sesame oil, 1 tablespoon rice wine vinegar, ¼ teaspoon grated fresh ginger, and ⅛ teaspoon salt.

- Two small 2-to-3-inch diameter brown rice cakes.

- Cabbage Salad: 1 cup shredded cabbage dressed with a dressing made of 1 teaspoon miso, 1 teaspoon rice wine vinegar, and ¼ teaspoon honey.

- ¾ cup diced honeydew melon.

2,000 CALORIES/DAY: Make Edamame Dip with 1¼ cup cooked shelled edamame, 2½ teaspoons sesame oil, 1 tablespoon rice wine vinegar, ¼ teaspoon grated fresh ginger, and a pinch salt. Serve with four small 2-to-3-inch diameter brown rice cakes, Cabbage Salad, and 1 cup diced honeydew melon.

2,500 CALORIES/DAY: Serve Edamame Dip, rice cakes, and Cabbage Salad from 2,000 calories/day with 1½ cups diced honeydew melon with 1 tablespoon slivered almonds.

Dinner

1,500 AND 1,700 CALORIES/DAY:

- 1 serving Braised Chicken Legs in Red Wine with Lentils, Fennel, and Kale (page 257).

- 2 cups mixed greens and ¾ cup sliced raw white button mushrooms dressed with 1½ teaspoons olive oil, 1 tablespoon lemon juice, and 2 tablespoons fresh chives.

- 1¼ cups blueberries.

2,000 CALORIES/DAY: 1 serving Braised Chicken Legs in Red Wine with Lentils, Fennel, and Kale and mixed greens from above with a 1-ounce whole wheat roll and 1¾ cups blueberries.

2,500 CALORIES/DAY: 1 serving Braised Chicken Legs in Red Wine with Lentils, Fennel, and Kale and mixed greens from above using 2 teaspoons olive oil in dressing with two 1-ounce crusty whole wheat rolls and 1¾ cups blueberries.

Snack

ALL CALORIE LEVELS:

- 1 Acai Popsicle (page 269).

2,500 CALORIES/DAY EXTRA SNACK: Trail mix: 1 ounce whole wheat crackers (about 19 reduced-fat Wheat Thins), 1 tablespoon plus 2 teaspoons chopped pecans, and 1 tablespoon dark chocolate chips.

Treat

1,500 CALORIES/DAY: Omit the treat.

1,700 CALORIES/DAY:

- 3½ cups air-popped popcorn with 1 teaspoon olive oil, three spritzes of olive oil cooking spray, a dash of salt, and a dash of cayenne pepper.

2,000 CALORIES/DAY: 5 cups air popped popcorn with 1 teaspoon olive oil, five spritzes of olive oil cooking spray, a dash of salt, and a dash of cayenne pepper.

2,500 CALORIES/DAY: 6 cups air-popped popcorn with 1½ teaspoons olive oil, five spritzes of olive oil cooking spray, a dash of salt, and a dash of cayenne pepper.

Day 4

Breakfast

1,500 CALORIES/DAY:

- 6 tablespoons Irish oatmeal cooked with water and topped with 1 tablespoon dried apricots and 1 tablespoon almonds.

- 1 cup skim milk.

1,700, 2,000, AND 2,500 CALORIES/DAY: 6 tablespoons Irish oatmeal cooked with water and topped with 2 tablespoons dried apricots, 1½ tablespoons almonds, and 1 cup skim milk.

Lunch

1,500 AND 1,700 CALORIES/DAY:

- 6 pieces store- or restaurant-bought salmon and avocado sushi roll.

- ¾ cup fresh pineapple chunks topped with 1 tablespoon plus 1 teaspoon chopped walnuts.

2,000 CALORIES/DAY: 9 pieces store- or restaurant-bought salmon and avocado sushi roll served with ¾ cup fresh pineapple chunks topped with 1 tablespoon plus 1 teaspoon chopped walnuts.

2,500 CALORIES/DAY: 9 pieces salmon and avocado sushi roll served with 1 cup fresh pineapple chunks topped with 2½ tablespoons chopped walnuts.

Dinner

1,500 AND 1,700 CALORIES/DAY:

- 1 serving Slow-Cooked Lamb with Tomato, Cauliflower, and Chard (page 261).

- Whole Grain Crostini: Brush two medium slices of whole grain bread (150 calories' worth or 1.6 ounces total) with 2 teaspoons olive oil. Place in a warm oven or toaster oven until slightly browned and crispy.

- 1 large orange

2,000 CALORIES/DAY: 1 serving Lamb served with Whole Grain Crostini and 1 large orange, sectioned and mixed with 1 cup blueberries and 2 teaspoons macadamia nuts.

2,500 CALORIES/DAY: 1 serving Lamb served with Whole Grain Crostini prepared with 1 tablespoon olive oil, plus 1 large orange, sectioned and mixed with 1½ cups blueberries and 1 tablespoon macadamia nuts.

Snack

ALL CALORIE LEVELS:

- ½ cup nonfat plain yogurt with ½ cup raspberries and 1 teaspoon cashews mixed in and ½ graham cracker (one square) crumbled on top.

2,500 CALORIES/DAY EXTRA SNACK: 2 Wasa multigrain crispbreads, sprinkled with 1½ tablespoons reduced-fat mozzarella cheese and 2 tablespoons chopped tomato. Heat in the toaster oven until cheese melts, about 1 minute. Serve with ¾ cup grapes.

Treat

1,500 CALORIES/DAY: Omit the treat.

1,700 CALORIES/DAY:

- 1 large banana sliced and topped with 12 regular-size dark chocolate chips and 1 teaspoon pine nuts.

2,000 CALORIES/DAY: ½ medium banana, sliced, and ¾ cup pear slices topped with 36 regular-size dark chocolate chips and 2 teaspoons pine nuts.

2,500 CALORIES/DAY: ½ medium banana, sliced, and 1 cup pear slices topped with 36 regular-size dark chocolate chips and 1 tablespoon plus 1 teaspoon pine nuts.

Day 5

Breakfast

1,500 CALORIES/DAY:

- Blackberry Smoothie: In a blender puree until smooth, 1 cup frozen blackberries, ½ medium frozen banana (peel banana, place in a sealed plastic bag, and freeze), 1½ tablespoons peanut butter, and ¾ cup plain nonfat yogurt.

1,700, 2,000, AND 2,500 CALORIES/DAY: Make Blackberry Smoothie with 1 cup frozen blackberries, ½ large frozen banana, 1½ tablespoons peanut butter, and 1 cup plain nonfat yogurt.

Lunch

1,500 AND 1,700 CALORIES/DAY:

- 1¹/₂ cups canned lentil soup (no more than 300 mg sodium per 1½ cup serving, such as Health Valley Organic no salt added lentil soup). Add 2 cups baby spinach and 2 teaspoons Parmesan cheese to soup while heating.

- 1 Wasa multigrain crispbread spread with 1 teaspoon Bestlife spread.

- ½ grapefruit, sectioned and topped with 2 tablespoons pistachios.

2,000 CALORIES/DAY: Serve 2 cups lentil soup with 2 cups baby spinach and 2 teaspoons Parmesan cheese added to soup while heating, one Wasa multigrain crispbread spread with 1 teaspoon Bestlife spread, and one grapefruit, sectioned and topped with 3 tablespoons pistachios.

2,500 CALORIES/DAY: Serve 2 cups canned lentil soup with 2 cups baby spinach and 2 teaspoons Parmesan cheese added to soup while heating, two Wasa multigrain crispbreads each spread with 1 teaspoon Bestlife spread, and one grapefruit, sectioned and drizzled with ½ teaspoon honey and 2½ tablespoons pistachios.

Dinner

1,500 AND 1,700 CALORIES/DAY:

- 1 serving Spiced Cod (page 263).

- Cracked Wheat Salad: ⅔ cup cooked cracked wheat (bulgur) prepared according to package directions, combined with ⅛ teaspoon salt, ¼ cup fresh pomegranate seeds (substitute 1 cup orange sections for pomegranate seeds if not available), 1 tablespoon olive oil, 2 tablespoons chopped mint, and 2 tablespoons chopped parsley.

2,000 CALORIES/DAY: 1 serving Spiced Cod served with Cracked Wheat Salad prepared with 1 cup plus 2 tablespoons cooked cracked wheat (bulgur) combined with ⅛ teaspoon salt, 5 tablespoons fresh pomegranate seeds, or 1½ cups orange sections, 1 tablespoon olive oil, 2 tablespoons chopped mint, and 2 tablespoons chopped parsley.

2,500 CALORIES/DAY: 1 serving Spiced Cod served with Cracked Wheat Salad prepared with 1¼ cups cooked cracked wheat combined with ⅛ teaspoon salt, 6 tablespoons fresh pomegranate seeds or 1½ cups orange sections, 1 tablespoon plus 1 teaspoon olive oil, 2 tablespoons chopped mint, and 2 tablespoons chopped parsley.

Snack

ALL CALORIE LEVELS:

- 1 Acai Popsicle (page 269).

2,500 CALORIES/DAY EXTRA SNACK: 1 small, 4-inch whole wheat pita, spread with 2 tablespoons sunflower seed butter.

Treat

1,500 CALORIES/DAY: Omit the treat.

1,700 CALORIES/DAY:

- Pretzels, Golden Raisins, and Dark Chocolate Trail Mix: 50 calories' worth or about ½ ounce pretzels combined with 2½ tablespoons golden raisins and 2 teaspoons or about 15 regular-size dark chocolate chips.

2,000 CALORIES/DAY: Pretzels, Golden Raisins, and Dark Chocolate Trail Mix prepared with 50 calories' worth or about ½ ounce pretzels with 3 tablespoons golden raisins and 1 tablespoon plus 1 teaspoon or about 30 regular-size dark chocolate chips.

2,500 CALORIES/DAY: Pretzels, Golden Raisins, and Dark Chocolate Trail Mix prepared with 75 calories' worth or about ¾ ounce pretzels with 4 tablespoons golden raisins and 1 tablespoon plus 1 teaspoon or about 30 regular-size dark chocolate chips.

Day 6

Breakfast

1,500 CALORIES/DAY:

- Yogurt Parfait: In a medium-size bowl, combine ⅔ cup plain nonfat yogurt, 2 crushed Wasa multigrain crispbreads, ½ banana, sliced, ¾ cup blueberries, and 2 tablespoons roughly chopped walnuts. Let sit overnight or serve immediately.

1,700, 2,000, AND 2,500 CALORIES/DAY: Yogurt Parfait prepared with ¾ cup plain nonfat yogurt, 2 crushed Wasa multigrain crispbreads, 2 teaspoons honey, ½ banana, sliced, ¾ cup blueberries, and 2 tablespoons roughly chopped walnuts.

Lunch

1,500 AND 1,700 CALORIES/DAY:

- Cannellini Bean Spread on Whole Grain Pita: In a food processor, combine until smooth ¾ cup cannellini beans (cooked or canned, no salt added, drained and rinsed), 2½ teaspoons olive oil, a dash of salt, 2 tablespoons fresh basil, and 2 tablespoons water. Spread mixture in a small (4-inch diameter) whole grain pita bread and add a slice of tomato.

- Arugula Salad: 2 cups of arugula dressed with ½ teaspoon olive oil and fresh lemon juice to taste.

- ½ cup cubed honeydew melon.

2,000 CALORIES/DAY: Cannellini Bean Spread on Whole Grain Pita prepared with 1 cup cannellini beans, 1 tablespoon olive oil, a dash of salt, 2 tablespoons fresh basil, and 2 tablespoons water. Spread in a small (4-inch diameter) whole grain pita bread with a slice of tomato. Serve with Arugula Salad and ¾ cup cubed honeydew topped with 1 tablespoon pistachios.

2,500 CALORIES/DAY: Cannellini Bean Spread on Whole Grain Pita with Tomato and Arugula Salad as prepared in 2,000 calories/day, and served with 1⅓ cups cubed honeydew topped with 2 tablespoons pistachios.

Dinner

1,500 AND 1,700 CALORIES/DAY:

- 1 serving Sweet Potato and Turkey Shepherd's Pie (page 260).

- Cole Slaw with Mustard Vinaigrette: 1 cup sliced cabbage with a dressing made of 2 teaspoons cider vinegar, 2 teaspoons olive oil, ¼ teaspoon mustard powder, 1 teaspoon honey, a pinch of salt, and cayenne pepper if desired.

- 1-ounce (about 73 calories) whole wheat roll served with 1 teaspoon olive oil mixed with 2 teaspoons of chopped basil for dipping.

- ¾ cup raspberries.

2,000 CALORIES/DAY: 1 serving Sweet Potato and Turkey Shepherd's Pie served with Cole Slaw and a 1-ounce whole wheat roll served with 2½ teaspoons olive oil mixed with 2 teaspoons chopped basil for dipping. Serve with 1½ cups raspberries, drizzled with ½ teaspoon honey and 1 teaspoon pomegranate seeds.

2,500 CALORIES/DAY: 1 serving Sweet Potato and Turkey Shepherd's Pie served with Cole Slaw and a 1-ounce whole wheat roll served with 2½ teaspoons olive oil mixed with 2 teaspoons chopped basil for dipping. Serve with 1½ cups raspberries, drizzled with 2 teaspoons honey and 1 tablespoon pomegranate seeds.

Snack

ALL CALORIE LEVELS:

- Strawberry Milk: 1¼ cups cold vanilla-flavored soy milk blended until smooth with ½ cup sliced fresh strawberries.

2,500 CALORIES/DAY EXTRA SNACK: 1 small sliced pear spread with 1 tablespoon plus 2 teaspoons almond butter.

Treat

1,500 CALORIES/DAY: Omit the treat.

1,700 CALORIES/DAY:

- 1 serving Baked Apple (page 271).

2,000 CALORIES/DAY: 1 serving Baked Apple topped with ½ ounce or
1 tablespoon low-fat caramel sauce and ½ teaspoon pecans.

2,500 CALORIES/DAY: 1 serving Baked Apple topped with ½ ounce or
1 tablespoon low-fat caramel sauce and 1 tablespoon pecans.

Day 7

Breakfast

1,500 CALORIES/DAY:

- Banana Spice Smoothie: In a blender combine until smooth 1 medium
  frozen banana (peel banana, place in a sealed plastic bag, and freeze),
  1 tablespoon ground flaxseed, ½ cup silken tofu, pinch of cinnamon,
  pinch of nutmeg, and 1¼ cups soy milk.

- 1 Wasa multigrain crispbread.

1,700, 2,000, AND 2,500 CALORIES/DAY: Banana Spice Smoothie as above;
spread 2 teaspoons peanut butter on the Wasa multigrain crispbread.

Lunch

1,500 AND 1,700 CALORIES/DAY:

- Goat Cheese Sandwich: Spread one toasted 1-ounce slice of whole grain
  bread with ½ ounce goat cheese, layer with 2 large slices tomato and
  ½ cup chopped purslane (if you cannot find purslane, use watercress
  or arugula).

- Citrus Salad: 1 cup orange and 1 cup grapefruit sections with
  3 tablespoons sunflower seeds.

2,000 CALORIES/DAY: Prepare Goat Cheese Sandwich with two toasted
1-ounce slices of whole grain bread and the Citrus Salad from above with
⅔ cup grapes added.

2,500 CALORIES/DAY: Goat Cheese Sandwich as prepared for 2,000 calories/ day and the Citrus Salad with 1 cup grapes and 2 teaspoons of maple syrup added.

Dinner

1,500 AND 1,700 CALORIES/DAY:

- 1 serving Trout Gumbo (page 264).

- Mixed Baby Green Salad: 2 cups greens with 1 teaspoon olive oil, a dash of salt, and a splash of lemon juice.

- ¾ cup raspberries.

2,000 CALORIES/DAY: 1 serving Trout Gumbo with the Mixed Baby Green Salad, ⅓ cup cooked brown rice prepared according to package directions seasoned with 1 teaspoon olive oil, a dash of salt, and 2 tablespoons finely chopped fresh parsley, and ¾ cup raspberries.

2,500 CALORIES/DAY: 1 serving Trout Gumbo with the Mixed Baby Green Salad, ¾ cup cooked brown rice seasoned with 1 teaspoon olive oil, a dash of salt, and 2 tablespoons finely chopped fresh parsley, and ¾ cup raspberries.

Snack

ALL CALORIE LEVELS:

- Cucumber with Yogurt Dip: In a small bowl thoroughly combine ¾ cup nonfat plain yogurt, ½ teaspoon olive oil, 1 teaspoon fresh-squeezed lemon juice, and ¼ teaspoon finely chopped chives. Serve with 1 cup cucumber slices.

2,500 CALORIES/DAY EXTRA SNACK: Spread 1½ tablespoons peanut butter on two Wasa multigrain crispbreads and sprinkle with 1 tablespoon thinly sliced celery and ½ teaspoon honey.

Treat

1,500 CALORIES/DAY: Omit the treat.

1,700 CALORIES/DAY:

- ¹/₂ cup plus 2 tablespoons dark chocolate sorbet.

2,000 CALORIES/DAY: Top the sorbet with 2 teaspoons chopped pecans.

2,500 CALORIES/DAY: Top the sorbet with 1½ tablespoons chopped pecans.

Day 8

Breakfast

1,500 CALORIES/DAY:

- Yogurt Pomegranate Parfait: ²/₃ cup nonfat plain yogurt with 2 tablespoons pomegranate seeds (substitute 2½ tablespoons dried apricots, chopped, or ¾ cup raspberries if pomegranate is not available), ½ cup blackberries, and 1 tablespoon chopped walnuts mixed in.

- 1 whole wheat English muffin toasted and spread with 2 teaspoons Bestlife spread.

1,700, 2,000, AND 2,500 CALORIES/DAY: Prepare parfait with 2 tablespoons walnuts. Serve with English muffin prepared as above.

Lunch

1,500 AND 1,700 CALORIES/DAY:

- Couscous Peach Salad: 1 cup cooked whole wheat couscous tossed with ½ cup sliced peaches, ¼ cup chickpeas from a can, drained and rinsed, and 1 tablespoon pine nuts, dressed with 1 teaspoon olive oil, 2 teaspoons sherry vinegar, a dash of salt, and black pepper to taste.

- Quick Roasted Kale: Heat oven to 350 degrees. Place 2 cups thinly sliced kale on a tray and lightly coat with vegetable oil spray, a dash of salt, and black pepper. Cook for 5 minutes, stirring often. After 5 minutes add 1 tablespoon balsamic vinegar, return to oven, and cook for an additional 2 minutes.

2,000 CALORIES/DAY: Prepare Couscous Peach Salad with 1 cup whole wheat couscous tossed with 1 cup sliced peaches, ⅓ cup chickpeas and 1 tablespoon pine nuts, dressed with 1 tablespoon olive oil, 2 teaspoons sherry vinegar, a dash of salt, and black pepper to taste. Serve with Quick Roasted Kale.

2,500 CALORIES/DAY: Prepare Couscous Peach Salad from 2,000 calories/day lunch with 2 tablespoons of pine nuts, and add 1 teaspoon olive oil to the Quick Roasted Kale.

Dinner

1,500 AND 1,700 CALORIES/DAY:

- 1 serving Creamy Mac and No Cheese (page 266).

- Tomato Salad: 1 large tomato cut into wedges with ¼ cup very thinly sliced red onion, dressed with 2 teaspoons olive oil and a splash red wine vinegar.

- Steamed Broccoli with Garlic: Place 1 cup of broccoli florets and 1 clove of finely minced garlic in a small saucepan. Add ¼ cup of water, cover, and cook until broccoli is tender, about 3 minutes. Drain and dress with 1 teaspoon olive oil and ⅛ teaspoon salt.

2,000 CALORIES/DAY: 1 serving Creamy Mac and No Cheese, Tomato Salad, and Steamed Broccoli with Garlic prepared with 1 tablespoon olive oil.

2,500 CALORIES/DAY: 1 serving Creamy Mac and No Cheese, Tomato Salad with the addition of ½ of a chopped avocado, and Steamed Broccoli with Garlic prepared the same way as the 2,000 calories/day.

Snack

ALL CALORIE LEVELS:

- Grape, Cardamom, and Yogurt Parfait: ¾ cup nonfat plain yogurt with ⅓ cup grapes, 2 teaspoons pumpkin seeds, and ½ teaspoon cardamom.

2,500 CALORIES/DAY EXTRA SNACK: 2 Wasa multigrain crispbreads each spread with 2½ teaspoons tahini and topped with 1 tablespoon shredded carrot.

Treat

1,500 CALORIES/DAY: Omit the treat.

1,700 CALORIES/DAY:

- 1 serving Chocolate Sesame Biscotti (page 271).

2,000 CALORIES/DAY: Chocolate Sesame Biscotti spread with 2 teaspoons almond butter.

2,500 CALORIES/DAY: Chocolate Sesame Biscotti spread with 1 tablespoon almond butter.

Day 9

Breakfast

1,500 CALORIES/DAY:

- Tofu Scramble: Heat a heavy-bottom skillet over medium heat and add 2 teaspoons olive oil. Add 1 tablespoon of finely chopped onion, then crumble 6 ounces firm tofu (if possible, buy tofu with a label that notes it's been processed with calcium sulfate) into the pan. Cook, stirring often, for 5 minutes. Season with ⅛ teaspoon salt. Serve rolled in an 8-inch diameter whole grain tortilla with ½ cup diced tomato and minced fresh hot pepper to taste.

- ½ cup sliced fresh mango and ½ cup blackberries.

1,700, 2,000, AND 2,500 CALORIES/DAY: Prepare Tofu Scramble using 1 tablespoon of olive oil. Serve with mango and blackberries as above.

Lunch

1,500 AND 1,700 CALORIES/DAY:

- Open-Face Almond Butter Sandwich: Spread one 1-ounce slice whole wheat bread with 1 tablespoon almond butter and top with ¼ cup roughly chopped dried figs and ⅓ cup roughly chopped grapes.

- Celery Salad: 1½ cups sliced celery dressed with 2½ teaspoons olive oil, ½ teaspoon fresh lemon juice, and ½ teaspoon Dijon mustard.

2,000 CALORIES/DAY: Prepare Almond Butter Sandwiches with two 1-ounce slices of whole wheat bread spread with 1 tablespoon plus 2 teaspoons almond butter and topped with ¼ cup roughly chopped dried figs and ½ cup roughly chopped grapes. Serve with Celery Salad.

2,500 CALORIES/DAY: Prepare Almond Butter Sandwiches with two 1-ounce slices of whole wheat bread spread with 2 tablespoons almond butter and topped with ⅓ cup roughly chopped dried figs and ⅔ cup roughly chopped grapes. Serve with Celery Salad.

Dinner

1,500 AND 1,700 CALORIES/DAY:

- 1 serving Salmon Salad with Avocado, Hijiki, Cucumber, and Mushrooms (page 264).

- ⅓ cup black rice (use brown if black not available) cooked according to package directions and seasoned with 1 teaspoon sesame oil, ⅛ teaspoon salt, and 2 tablespoons chopped fresh cilantro.

- ½ grapefruit and ½ cup raspberries.

2,000 CALORIES/DAY: 1 serving Salmon Salad and ⅔ cup black rice seasoned with 1 teaspoon sesame oil, ⅛ teaspoon salt, and 2 tablespoons chopped fresh cilantro. Serve with a whole grapefruit sprinkled with 2 teaspoons chopped walnuts.

2,500 CALORIES/DAY: 1 serving Salmon Salad and 1 cup black rice seasoned with 1 teaspoon sesame oil, ⅛ teaspoon salt, and 2 tablespoons chopped fresh cilantro. Serve with a whole grapefruit sprinkled with 1 tablespoon chopped walnuts.

Snack

ALL CALORIE LEVELS:

- 1 green tea bag steeped in 1½ cups hot soy milk.

2,500 CALORIES/DAY EXTRA SNACK: 1 large banana sliced lengthwise and spread with 1½ tablespoons sunflower seed butter.

Treat

1,500 CALORIES/DAY: Omit the treat.

1,700 CALORIES/DAY:

- Poached Pear: Peel pear, slice in half, and core. In a saucepan deep enough to accommodate the pear, bring 2 cups of water and 2 tablespoons of sugar to a boil. Add 1 tablespoon of lemon zest, a whole vanilla bean cut in half lengthwise, and the pear. Reduce heat to simmer and cook until tender, 20–30 minutes depending on variety of the pear. Serve drizzled with 2 tablespoons nonfat sour cream, 1 teaspoon honey, and 2 tablespoons of the poaching liquid.

2,000 CALORIES/DAY: Poached Pear served with 1 tablespoon chopped pecans.

2,500 CALORIES/DAY: Poached Pear served with 2 tablespoons chopped pecans.

Day 10

Breakfast

1,500 CALORIES/DAY:

- Egg White and Spinach Omelet: Prepared with 2 egg whites, 1 tablespoon reduced-fat feta cheese, and 2 cups spinach. Use 2½ teaspoons olive oil for cooking.

- 1 Wasa multigrain crispbread.

- 1 cup blackberries drizzled with 1 teaspoon honey.

- 1 cup skim milk.

1,700, 2,000, AND 2,500 CALORIES/DAY: Egg White and Spinach Omelet served with one Wasa multigrain crispbread, 1½ cups blackberries drizzled with 2 teaspoons honey, and 1 cup skim milk.

Lunch

1,500 AND 1,700 CALORIES/DAY:

- Portobello Sandwich: 1 portobello mushroom rubbed with 1 teaspoon olive oil and baked in a 350-degree oven until tender, about 20 minutes, served on a 1½-ounce whole grain bun with 1 slice of red onion and a slice of tomato.

- 1 sliced plum tossed with 1 teaspoon olive oil, a splash of red wine, and 1½ tablespoons roughly chopped pistachios.

- 10 baby carrots dipped into 2 teaspoons tahini.

2,000 CALORIES/DAY: Portobello Sandwich prepared as above using 1½ teaspoons olive oil, served with 1 sliced plum tossed with 1 teaspoon olive oil, a splash of red wine, and 3 tablespoons roughly chopped pistachios, and 15 baby carrots dipped into 4 teaspoons tahini.

2,500 CALORIES/DAY: Portobello Sandwich prepared as above using 2 teaspoons olive oil, served with 1 sliced plum tossed with 1 teaspoon olive oil, a splash of red wine, and 3 tablespoons roughly chopped pistachios, and 25 baby carrots dipped into 1½ tablespoons tahini.

Dinner

1,500 AND 1,700 CALORIES/DAY:

- 1 serving Tofu Vegetable Soup with Kombu (page 267).

- 1 serving Whole Grain Thin Spaghetti with Peanut Sauce (page 268).

- 1 large orange.

2,000 CALORIES/DAY: 1 serving Tofu Vegetable Soup with Kombu and Whole Grain Thin Spaghetti with Peanut Sauce served with 1 large orange and 2 Wasa multigrain crispbreads spread with 1 teaspoon each Bestlife spread.

2,500 CALORIES/DAY: 1 serving Tofu Vegetable Soup with Kombu and Whole Grain Thin Spaghetti with Peanut Sauce served with 1 large orange and ¾ cup sliced strawberries and 3 Wasa multigrain crispbreads spread with 1 teaspoon each Bestlife spread.

Snack

ALL CALORIE LEVELS:

- Chocolate Ginger Latte: Steep 1 ginger tea bag in 1 cup of soy milk, then whisk in 2 teaspoons cocoa powder and 2 teaspoons sugar.

2,500 CALORIES/DAY EXTRA SNACK: Trail mix: 3 tablespoons toasted pine nuts and 15 reduced-fat Wheat Thins or 90 calories of your favorite whole grain cracker.

Treat

1,500 CALORIES/DAY: Omit the treat.

1,700 CALORIES/DAY:

- Orange with Spices and Pecans: Toss sections of one medium orange, peel and pith removed, with a pinch of cinnamon, cardamom, and powdered ginger. Top with 1½ tablespoons chopped pecans.

2,000 CALORIES/DAY: Orange with Spices and Pecans prepared with 2 tablespoons plus 2 teaspoons chopped pecans.

2,500 CALORIES/DAY: Orange with Spices and Pecans prepared with 3 tablespoons chopped pecans.

Day 11

Breakfast

1,500 CALORIES/DAY:

- Whole Grain Cream of Wheat: 3 tablespoons Healthy Grain Instant Original Cream of Wheat cooked according to package instructions with 1 medium apple, shredded, ¼ teaspoon cinnamon, ½ cup raspberries, 2 teaspoons ground flaxseed, and 1½ tablespoons chopped walnuts.

- 1 cup skim milk.

1,700, 2,000, AND 2,500 CALORIES/DAY: Healthy Grain Instant Original Cream of Wheat prepared as above served with ¾ cup raspberries, 1 tablespoon ground flaxseed, and 2 tablespoons chopped walnuts. Serve with 1 cup skim milk.

Lunch

1,500 AND 1,700 CALORIES/DAY:

- 1 serving Sesame Shrimp Salad with Napa Cabbage and Bean Sprouts (page 256).

- 1 cup blueberries topped with 2 tablespoons nonfat plain yogurt.

2,000 CALORIES/DAY: 1 serving Sesame Shrimp Salad served with 1 brown rice cake spread with ¼ avocado, mashed, and 1 cup blueberries topped with 2 tablespoons nonfat plain yogurt.

2,500 CALORIES/DAY: 1 serving Sesame Shrimp Salad served with 2 brown rice cakes spread with ⅓ avocado, mashed, and 1 cup blueberries topped with 2 tablespoons nonfat plain yogurt.

Dinner

1,500 AND 1,700 CALORIES/DAY:

- 1 serving Veggie Chili with Kale (page 268).

- 1 serving Polenta (page 269).

2,000 CALORIES/DAY: 1 serving Veggie Chili with Kale and Polenta with 2 tablespoons (½ ounce) reduced-fat cheddar cheese melted on the polenta. Add salad of 2 cups mixed baby greens with ½ cup sliced white button mushrooms, 1 medium tomato, chopped, 1 teaspoon olive oil, and a splash of red wine vinegar.

2,500 CALORIES/DAY: 1 serving Veggie Chili with Kale and Polenta prepared as for 2,000 calories/day. Prepare the salad with 2 teaspoons olive oil.

Snack

ALL CALORIE LEVELS:

- Grape, Cinnamon, and Yogurt Parfait: ⅔ cup plain nonfat yogurt with ½ cup grapes and ¼ teaspoon ground cinnamon.

2,500 CALORIES/DAY EXTRA SNACK: 3½ tablespoons sunflower seeds with ¼ cup pomegranate seeds.

Treat

1,500 CALORIES/DAY: Omit the treat.

1,700 CALORIES/DAY:

- Dark Chocolate with Fresh Strawberries: 1¼ cups whole strawberries with 12 regular-size dark chocolate chips and 1 tablespoon plus 1 teaspoon chopped pecans.

2,000 CALORIES/DAY: Prepare Dark Chocolate with Fresh Strawberries with 1¼ cups whole strawberries and 36 regular-size dark chocolate chips and 1 tablespoon plus 2 teaspoons chopped pecans.

2,500 CALORIES/DAY: Prepare Dark Chocolate with Fresh Strawberries with 1 cup whole strawberries with 48 regular-size dark chocolate chips and 3 tablespoons chopped pecans.

Day 12

Breakfast

1,500 CALORIES/DAY:

- ¼ cup dry steel-cut oats cooked according to package directions in 1 cup soy milk with 1 vanilla bean sliced lengthwise or ⅛ teaspoon vanilla extract, and topped with ¾ cup chopped fresh strawberries and 2 tablespoons slivered almonds.

1,700, 2,000, AND 2,500 CALORIES/DAY: ¼ cup dry steel-cut oats cooked according to package directions in 1 cup soy milk with 1 vanilla bean sliced lengthwise or ⅛ teaspoon vanilla extract, and topped with ¾ cup chopped fresh strawberries and 3 tablespoons slivered almonds.

Lunch

1,500 AND 1,700 CALORIES/DAY:

- Tempeh, Lettuce and Tomato Sandwich: Preheat oven to broil. In a food processor combine ¼ avocado, a pinch of salt, and 1 tablespoon silken tofu. Set aside. Place a 4-ounce slice of tempeh in the oven and cook on each side for 3 minutes. Toast two 1-ounce slices of whole grain bread and spread each with ½ of the avocado mixture, top with tempeh, a slice of tomato, and two leaves of romaine lettuce.

2,000 CALORIES/DAY: Prepare sandwich as above using ½ avocado, a pinch of salt, and 2 tablespoons silken tofu, a 4½-ounce slice of tempeh, two 1-ounce slices of whole grain bread, a slice of tomato, and two leaves of romaine lettuce. Serve with a salad of 2 cups spinach leaves topped with a splash of balsamic vinegar and ½ teaspoon olive oil.

2,500 CALORIES/DAY: Prepare sandwich and spinach salad as 2,000 calories/ day. Serve with 1¼ cups sliced peaches.

Dinner

1,500 AND 1,700 CALORIES/DAY:

- 1 serving Poached Chicken Curry (page 258) garnished with 1 tablespoon reduced-fat sour cream.

- ¼ cup cooked brown rice seasoned with 1 teaspoon olive oil and a dash of salt.

2,000 CALORIES/DAY: 1 serving Poached Chicken Curry garnished with 1 tablespoon reduced-fat sour cream and served with ⅓ cup cooked brown rice seasoned with 2½ teaspoons olive oil, a dash of salt, and Spicy Mango Relish: ⅓ cup mango cubes combined with chopped fresh hot pepper to taste, 2 tablespoons chopped fresh cilantro, and a pinch of salt.

2,500 CALORIES/DAY: 1 serving Poached Chicken Curry garnished with 1 tablespoon reduced-fat sour cream and served with ⅔ cup cooked brown rice seasoned with 2½ teaspoons olive oil and a dash of salt. Prepare Spicy Mango Relish with ½ cup mango cubes.

Snack

ALL CALORIE LEVELS:

- Cucumber with Ricotta Dip: ⅓ cup plus 2 tablespoons nonfat ricotta cheese mixed with a pinch of paprika, 1 tablespoon plus 1 teaspoon cashews, and ⅛ teaspoon fresh lemon juice with 1 cup sliced cucumber for dipping.

2,500 CALORIES/DAY EXTRA SNACK: 6 ounces nonfat Greek yogurt with 3 tablespoons peanuts and 24 regular-size dark chocolate chips.

Treat

1,500 CALORIES/DAY: Omit the treat.

1,700 CALORIES/DAY:

- 1 Carrot Oatmeal Cookie (page 272)

2,000 CALORIES/DAY: 1 Carrot Oatmeal Cookie spread with 1½ teaspoons almond butter.

2,500 CALORIES/DAY: 1 Carrot Oatmeal Cookie spread with 2½ teaspoons almond butter and topped with 1 teaspoon almonds.

Day 13

Breakfast

1,500 CALORIES/DAY:

- ¾ cup whole grain flake cereal (such as Arrowhead Mills Oat Bran Flakes, Nature's Path Flax Plus, or Kashi-7 Whole Grain Flakes) mixed with ½ cup Shredded Wheat.

- 2 teaspoons sunflower seeds

- ¾ cup blackberries

- 1 cup soy milk

1,700, 2,000, AND 2,500 CALORIES/DAY: 1 cup whole grain flake cereal mixed with ½ cup Shredded Wheat, 1 tablespoon sunflower seeds, ¾ cup blackberries, and 1 cup soy milk.

Lunch

1,500 AND 1,700 CALORIES/DAY:

- Tuna Salad: In a large bowl combine 4 ounces low-sodium chunk light tuna packed in water, drained, with 1 teaspoon capers, 1 medium tomato, diced, 1 teaspoon Dijon mustard, ½ cup sliced cucumbers, ½ cup sliced celery, 1 cup arugula, 2 teaspoons olive oil, and 1 teaspoon fresh lemon juice.

- 1 Wasa multigrain crispbread.

- 1 cup sliced strawberries.

2,000 CALORIES/DAY: Prepare Tuna Salad with 5 ounces tuna, 1 teaspoon capers, 1 medium tomato, diced, 1 teaspoon sesame seeds, 1 teaspoon Dijon mustard, ½ cup sliced cucumbers, ½ cup sliced celery, 1 cup arugula, 1 tablespoon olive oil, and 1 teaspoon fresh lemon juice. Serve with a 1-ounce whole wheat roll and 1 cup sliced strawberries.

2,500 CALORIES/DAY: Prepare Tuna Salad as for 2,000 calories/day. Serve with two 1-ounce whole wheat rolls and 1 cup sliced strawberries.

Dinner

1,500 AND 1,700 CALORIES/DAY:

- 1 serving Pork Tenderloin with Turnips, Apples, and Onions (page 262).

- 1 cup barley cooked according to package directions and combined with 2 teaspoons olive oil, 1 cup of arugula, one dash of salt, and black pepper to taste.

2,000 CALORIES/DAY: 1 serving Pork Tenderloin with Turnips, Apples, and Onions served with 1¼ cups barley combined with 1 tablespoon olive oil, 2 teaspoons chopped pecans, 1 cup of arugula, one dash of salt, and black pepper to taste.

2,500 CALORIES/DAY: 1 serving Pork Tenderloin with Turnips, Apples, and Onions served with 1½ cups barley combined with 1 tablespoon olive oil, 1 tablespoon plus 1 teaspoon chopped pecans, 1 cup of arugula, a dash of salt, and black pepper to taste.

Snack

ALL CALORIE LEVELS:

- Mango Smoothie: Combine in a blender until smooth ½ cup sliced fresh mango and 1 cup calcium-enriched soy milk.

2,500 CALORIES/DAY EXTRA SNACK: 10 rice crackers (about 115 calories' worth) dipped in 1 tablespoon plus 1 teaspoon tahini mixed with 1 tablespoon pomegranate seeds.

Treat

1,500 CALORIES/DAY: Omit the treat.

1,700 CALORIES/DAY:

- 1 serving Stuffed Baked Peach (page 272).

2,000 CALORIES/DAY: 1 serving Stuffed Baked Peach and ½ cup plain nonfat Greek yogurt.

2,500 CALORIES/DAY: 1 serving Stuffed Baked Peach and ¾ cup plain nonfat Greek yogurt topped with 1 teaspoon almonds.

Day 14

Breakfast

1,500 CALORIES/DAY:

- 1 serving Blueberry Oatmeal Pancakes with ¼ cup reserved blueberries included in recipe (page 256).

- ⅔ cup calcium-fortified orange juice.

1,700, 2,000, AND 2,500 CALORIES/DAY: 1 serving Blueberry Oatmeal Pancakes topped with ¼ cup reserved blueberries included in recipe and 2 teaspoons chopped walnuts. Serve with ¾ cup calcium-fortified orange juice.

Lunch

1,500 AND 1,700 CALORIES/DAY:

- Black Bean Salad: Toss 1 cup shredded cabbage with ½ cup cooked or canned (no salt, drained and rinsed) black beans, ½ cup sliced cucumber, 1 tablespoon finely chopped red onion, ¼ avocado sliced, 1 tablespoon fresh lime juice, 1½ teaspoons olive oil, ⅛ teaspoon salt, and black pepper to taste.

- Garlic Toast: Rub a 1-ounce slice of whole grain bread with ½ teaspoon olive oil and ⅛ teaspoon minced garlic, and toast under the broiler until golden brown.

- 1 orange.

2,000 CALORIES/DAY: Prepare Black Bean Salad as above but with 1 cup black beans. Serve with Garlic Toast and orange.

2,500 CALORIES/DAY: Prepare Black Bean Salad as 2,000 calories/day, and add one Wasa multigrain crispbread spread with 1½ teaspoons Bestlife spread. Serve with Garlic Toast and orange.

Dinner

1,500 AND 1,700 CALORIES/DAY:

- 1 serving Baked Penne Pasta with Shrimp (page 265).

- Arugula and Fennel Salad: 1 cup arugula and 1 cup finely shaved fennel dressed with 2 teaspoons olive oil, 1 teaspoon balsamic vinegar, a small pinch of salt, and black pepper to taste.

2,000 CALORIES/DAY: 1 serving Baked Penne Pasta with Shrimp and Arugula and Fennel Salad prepared with 2 cups arugula, 1 cup finely shaved fennel, ¼ cup grated carrot dressed with 1 tablespoon olive oil, 2 teaspoons balsamic vinegar, 1 tablespoon plus 1 teaspoon pine nuts, a small pinch of salt, and black pepper to taste.

2,500 CALORIES/DAY: 1 serving Baked Penne Pasta with Shrimp and Arugula and Fennel Salad prepared as for 2,000 calories/day. Serve with ¾ cup sliced apple drizzled with 2 teaspoons honey.

Snack

ALL CALORIE LEVELS:

- Carrots with Spiced Yogurt Dip: In a small bowl thoroughly combine ¾ cup nonfat plain yogurt, 1 teaspoon olive oil, a pinch of ground cumin, a pinch of cayenne pepper, ¼ teaspoon fennel seeds, and a pinch of salt. Serve with 6 medium carrot slices.

2,500 CALORIES/DAY EXTRA SNACK: 1 cup sliced green or yellow summer squash dipped into 6 tablespoons hummus mixed with 1 tablespoon plus 1 teaspoon toasted sesame seeds.

Treat

1,500 CALORIES/DAY: Omit the treat.

1,700 CALORIES/DAY:

- Trail mix: 2 teaspoons almonds, 3 tablespoons chopped dried figs, and 1 tablespoon cocoa nibs.

2,000 CALORIES/DAY: Prepare trail mix with 1 tablespoon almonds, 4 tablespoons chopped dried figs, and 1 tablespoon plus 1 teaspoon cocoa nibs.

2,500 CALORIES/DAY: Trail mix as prepared for 2,000 calories/day, served with 10 reduced-fat Wheat Thins or 60 calories of another whole wheat cracker.

20 YEARS YOUNGER RECIPES

Think of it as the best of both worlds: This collection of twenty-five recipes offers the anti-aging benefits of the Okinawan diet as well as those of Mediterranean traditions, with the distinctive flavors of each. Each recipe also contains one or more of the superfoods listed in chapter 3. Overall, they give you a lot of health rewards for your cooking efforts — and those efforts won't sap your energy: No recipe takes more than twenty minutes of preparation time. Enjoy!

Breakfast

MUESLI

Serves 4   Prep time: 5 minutes   Total time: 5 minutes

1½ cups rolled oats

¼ cup chopped dried fruits, such as apricots, prunes, or raisins (raisins can be left whole)

¼ cup chopped almonds

3 tablespoons raw pumpkin seeds

2 tablespoons ground flaxseed

½ teaspoon very finely chopped orange rind

1. Combine all ingredients in a medium bowl. Store any extra servings in an airtight container.

Per serving: 264 calories; 1.6 g saturated fat; 5 mg sodium; 6 g fiber

BLUEBERRY OATMEAL PANCAKES

Serves 4   Prep time: 5 minutes   Total time: 15 minutes

¾ cup spelt flour

⅓ cup plus 2 tablespoons wheat bran

⅓ cup plus 2 tablespoons oatmeal

½ teaspoon baking soda

½ cup egg substitute

1¾ cup buttermilk (more if batter is too thick)

1½ tablespoons canola oil

2 tablespoons Bestlife spread, melted

2 cups blueberries

Vegetable oil spray

1. Heat a heavy-bottom skillet over medium heat.

2. Mix spelt flour, bran, oatmeal, baking soda, egg substitute, buttermilk, oil, and Bestlife spread until just combined but a few lumps are still present. Do not overmix. Gently fold in 1 cup of the blueberries.

3. Spray hot skillet with cooking oil spray and drop batter onto skillet making 4 large or 8 small pancakes. When bubbles appear on the surface of the pancake, about 3 minutes, flip, and cook the other side for another 2 minutes.

4. Garnish with the remaining blueberries.

Per serving: 337 calories; 2.4 g saturated fat; 377 mg sodium; 8 g fiber

Lunch

SESAME SHRIMP SALAD WITH NAPA CABBAGE AND BEAN SPROUTS

Serves 4   Prep time: 10 minutes   Total time: 10 minutes

¼ cup sesame paste (tahini)

2 tablespoons rice wine vinegar

1 tablespoon water

¼ teaspoon salt

Hot pepper flakes, to taste

4 cups julienned Napa cabbage

1 cup bean sprouts

1 cup shredded carrots

1 pound shrimp, cooked and shelled

2 teaspoons sesame oil

Juice of 1 lemon

1. In a large bowl combine until smooth sesame paste, rice wine vinegar, water, salt, and hot pepper flakes. Add cabbage, bean sprouts, and carrots, and toss until thoroughly incorporated.

2. In a small bowl toss shrimp with sesame oil and lemon juice.

3. To serve, make a bed of cabbage mixture and top with the shrimp.

Per serving: 321 calories; 2 g saturated fat; 385 mg sodium; 4 g fiber

Dinner

BRAISED CHICKEN LEGS IN RED WINE WITH LENTILS, FENNEL, AND KALE

Serves 4   Prep time: 10 minutes   Total time: 1 hour

---

2 teaspoons olive oil	1 large sprig rosemary
4 chicken legs, skin removed	½ cup lentils
1 medium onion, finely chopped	1 cup sliced fennel
2 cloves garlic, finely chopped	2 cups chopped kale
1 cup red wine	¼ teaspoon salt
1 cup water	

1. Preheat oven to 325 degrees.

2. Heat a large ovenproof heavy-bottom pot with a lid over medium heat. Pour in olive oil and place legs in pot in a single layer and cook, turning once, until browned, about 10 minutes.

3. Remove legs and add onion and garlic to the pot. Cook, stirring often, for 3 minutes. Add wine, water, rosemary, and lentils, bring to a boil, then reduce heat and simmer for 5 minutes. Add chicken legs, fennel, and kale.

4. Cover pot and place in oven. Cook for 1 hour. Remove from oven, take out rosemary sprig, add salt, and serve.

Per serving: 331 calories; 3.8 g saturated fat; 255 mg sodium; 9 g fiber

Poached Chicken Curry

Serves 4   Prep time: 15 minutes   Total time: 45 minutes

1 tablespoon olive oil

1 onion, sliced

1 teaspoon cumin

1 teaspoon mustard powder

1 tablespoon minced fresh ginger

2 cloves garlic, minced

¼ teaspoon cayenne pepper, or to taste

2 large tomatoes, sliced, or 2 cups canned, no salt added

4 cups water

¼ teaspoon salt

Pepper, to taste

1 teaspoon turmeric

1 cup cooked garbanzo beans, dry or canned, no salt added, drained and rinsed

2 cups diced sweet potatoes

4 cups julienned collard greens

1 cup fresh or frozen peas

1 pound skinless, boneless chicken breasts, cut into ½-inch strips

1. Heat a heavy-bottom stockpot with a lid over medium heat. Add olive oil and onion to the pot. Cook, stirring often, for 5 minutes. Add cumin, mustard powder, ginger, garlic, and cayenne. Cook for 2 more minutes, stirring constantly.

2. Add tomatoes, water, salt, pepper, turmeric, garbanzo beans, sweet potatoes, and collard greens to the pot and bring to a boil. Reduce heat to a simmer and cook until the sweet potatoes are tender, about 20 minutes.

3. Add peas and chicken. Cover and simmer for 5 minutes, or until chicken is cooked through. Serve.

Per serving: 397 calories; 1.1 g saturated fat; 277 mg sodium; 11 g fiber

BAKED EGGPLANT AND GROUND TURKEY

Serves 4   Prep time: 20 minutes   Total time: 1 hour

4 cups thinly sliced eggplant	½ teaspoon cinnamon
1 onion, thinly sliced	½ teaspoon cumin
2 cloves garlic, minced	⅛ teaspoon salt
Vegetable oil cooking spray	Pepper to taste
12 ounces ground turkey	1 cup tomato sauce
1 tablespoon oregano	½ cup water

1. Preheat oven to 375 degrees. Heat a large heavy-bottom skillet over medium heat.

2. Coat eggplant, onion, and garlic with cooking spray. Place on a baking sheet and roast in oven for 15 minutes.

3. Spray turkey with cooking spray and cook in skillet, stirring often, until browned, about 5 minutes. Stir in oregano, cinnamon, cumin, salt, and pepper to taste.

4. Coat a 9×9-inch baking pan with cooking spray. Pour in ½ cup of the tomato sauce and top with half of the eggplant mixture, half of the turkey mixture, remaining eggplant mixture, remaining turkey mixture, and top with remaining tomato sauce. Pour the water around the edges.

5. Bake for 40 minutes. Serve hot.

Per serving: 206 calories; 2 g saturated fat; 387 mg sodium; 5 g fiber

Sweet Potato and Turkey Shepherd's Pie

Serves 4   Prep time: 20 minutes   Total time: 60 minutes

POTATOES

2 medium sweet potatoes

2 teaspoons olive oil

2 tablespoons skim milk

⅛ teaspoon salt

TURKEY

Vegetable oil cooking spray

2 large carrots, shredded

1 onion, chopped

1 pound boneless turkey tenderloin, chopped into 1-inch pieces

1 teaspoon fresh thyme

3 cups spinach

POTATOES

1. Preheat oven to 375 degrees. Cut potatoes in half lengthwise, place cut-side down in a baking pan, and bake in the oven until tender when tested with a fork, about 30 minutes.

2. Remove potatoes from the oven (leave the oven on), and scoop out the flesh. Place the flesh in a large bowl and add olive oil, milk, and salt and mash with a wooden spoon until smooth.

TURKEY MIXTURE (prepare while potatoes are cooking)

1. Heat a heavy-bottom skillet over medium heat.

2. Lightly coat skillet with cooking spray. Add carrots and onion and cook until slightly browned, about 4 minutes, stirring often.

3. Add turkey and thyme, cook until golden brown, about 5 minutes. Mix in spinach.

TO ASSEMBLE

1. In a 9×9-inch baking pan or four individual 4- or 5-inch ramekins, place turkey mixture on the bottom and cover with sweet potatoes.

2. Bake in a 375-degree oven for 15 minutes if using warm ingredients. (If you assembled pies earlier and refrigerated, bake about 25 minutes.)

3. After baking pies, turn oven to broil and broil 6 to 9 inches from heat source until tops of potatoes are browned, about 5 minutes. Serve hot.

Per serving: 239 calories; 1 g saturated fat; 212 mg sodium; 4 g fiber

SLOW-COOKED LAMB WITH TOMATO, CAULIFLOWER, AND CHARD

Serves 4   Prep time: 20 minutes   Total time: 2 hours

½ teaspoon cumin	1 onion, chopped
⅛ teaspoon cayenne	2 cloves of garlic, finely minced
¼ teaspoon turmeric	2 large tomatoes, chopped
½ teaspoon cinnamon	1 cup chopped cauliflower
1 pound boneless leg of lamb, cut into cubes	4 cups chard (or spinach if not available)
Vegetable oil cooking spray	¼ teaspoon salt
2 cups water	

1. In a large mixing bowl combine the cumin, cayenne, turmeric, and cinnamon. Add the lamb and toss until coated. Set aside.

2. Heat a large heavy-bottom pot with a lid over medium heat. Spray with vegetable oil and add half of the lamb, browning, about 3 minutes on each side. Remove the first batch of lamb and repeat with the remaining half. Remove the second batch of lamb and set aside.

3. Add the water and scrape the bottom of the pot to incorporate the spices stuck to the pot. Add the lamb, onion, garlic, and tomatoes.

4. Bring to a boil, reduce the heat to low, cover, and simmer for 1½ hours, stirring occasionally. Add the cauliflower and chard and cook for an additional 10 minutes. Add salt. Serve hot.

Per serving: 205 calories; 2.7 g saturated fat; 329 mg sodium; 3 g fiber

PORK TENDERLOIN WITH TURNIPS, APPLES, AND ONIONS

Serves 4   Prep time: 10 minutes   Total time: 2 hours

2 tablespoons paprika	½ teaspoon salt
1½ tablespoons olive oil	4 cloves garlic, minced
1 teaspoon ground cumin	1 pound pork tenderloin
1 tablespoon brown sugar	1 cup 1-inch cubes of turnip
1 tablespoon cocoa powder	1 cup 1-inch cubes of apple
1 tablespoon fresh oregano	1 onion, diced

1. Preheat oven to 325 degrees.

2. Blend paprika, 1 tablespoon of the oil, cumin, brown sugar, cocoa powder, oregano, salt, garlic, and 1 teaspoon water in food processor until it becomes a paste, about 1 minute.

3. Rub pork with mixture and allow to marinate in the refrigerator for 1 hour or up to 24 hours.

4. Place turnip, apple, and onion in a bowl and toss with remaining olive oil.

5. Place pork in baking pan and surround with turnip, apple, and onion. Bake until the internal temperature reaches 150 degrees (the temperature will rise while it is resting), about 45 minutes. Let rest for at least 10 minutes before slicing.

Per serving: 248 calories; 2 g saturated fat; 359 mg sodium; 4 g fiber

POACHED TROUT WITH TOMATO AND BASIL

Serves 4   Prep time: 10 minutes   Total time: 20 minutes

½ cup white wine	¼ cup basil leaves
1 large tomato, skin* and seeds removed, chopped	1 pound trout fillet, divided into 4 portions
1 cup water	⅛ teaspoon salt
2 tablespoons finely diced onion	

1. Place wine, tomato, water, onion, and basil in a heavy-bottom skillet (just large enough to fit fish so pieces do not overlap) and bring to a boil.

2. Reduce heat and let simmer for 5 minutes.

3. Add the trout, cover, and cook for an additional 5 minutes. Add salt.

4. Serve the fish in shallow bowls with the broth spooned on top.

   * To remove the skin of a tomato, dip it into boiling water for ten seconds, then place in a bowl of cold water. The skin should easily peel off.

Per serving: 150 calories; .8 g saturated fat; 112 mg sodium; 1 g fiber

SPICED COD

Serves 4   Prep time: 10 minutes   Total time: 25 minutes

1 tablespoon olive oil

2 cloves garlic, minced

¼ teaspoon cumin

¼ teaspoon turmeric

¼ teaspoon cinnamon

Crushed red pepper, to taste

4 large tomatoes, cores removed, and chopped

2 cups water

1 pound cod, cut into 4 portions

¼ teaspoon salt

1 lemon, cut into 4 wedges

1. Heat a large heavy-bottom skillet with a lid over medium heat. Add olive oil and garlic and cook, stirring constantly, for 1 minute.

2. Add cumin, turmeric, and cinnamon and cook for an additional 30 seconds, stirring constantly. Add red pepper, tomatoes, and water. Bring to a boil, then reduce heat to a simmer and cook for 10 minutes.

3. Add fish to spice broth, then cover and cook until fish flakes easily with a fork, about 4 minutes. Season with salt.

4. Serve fish with the spice broth and lemon wedges.

Per serving: 164 calories; .7 g saturated fat; 219 mg sodium; 3 g dietary fiber

Trout Gumbo

Serves 4   Prep time: 15 minutes   Total time: 55 minutes

1½ tablespoons olive oil

2 tablespoons all-purpose flour

1 tablespoon minced garlic

4 cups low-sodium vegetable broth

1 cup water

1 bottle beer

3 large tomatoes, chopped

1 onion, finely chopped

Fresh chili peppers, finely chopped, to taste

1 tablespoon Cajun seasoning

2 cups sliced okra (fresh or frozen)

1½ pounds trout fillet cut into 1-inch pieces

⅛ teaspoon salt

1. Heat a heavy-bottom pot over medium heat. Add oil and flour and whisk together until smooth. Cook, stirring constantly until browned and bubbly, about 5 minutes. Mix in garlic and cook for 1 minute.

2. Gradually add the vegetable broth, water, and beer, and combine thoroughly. Bring to a boil and mix in tomatoes, onion, chili peppers, Cajun seasoning, and okra. Reduce heat to a simmer, then cover and cook for 30 minutes, stirring often.

3. Add trout to soup and return to a simmer. Cover and cook until fish is flaky, about 5 minutes. Add salt and serve.

Per serving: 422 calories; 2.7 g saturated fat; 360 mg sodium; 5 g fiber

Salmon Salad with Avocado, Hijiki, Cucumber, and Mushrooms

Serves 4   Prep time: 15 minutes   Total time: 45 minutes

1 cup hijiki seaweed (if not available, substitute a green such as spinach, arugula, or watercress)

1½ pounds skinless center-cut salmon fillet (wild-caught, if possible)

¼ teaspoon salt

3 teaspoons sesame oil

1 lemon, halved

2 tablespoons rice wine vinegar

2 tablespoons finely chopped green onion

1 cup peeled, seeded and diced cucumber

1 cup sliced white button mushrooms

1 avocado, sliced

1. In a medium-size bowl pour enough warm water over the hijiki to cover and let stand for 30 minutes. (If using a green, skip this step.)

2. While the seaweed is soaking, cut the salmon in half lengthwise, then slice each piece crosswise into ¼-inch slices.

3. Fill a deep 10-inch skillet with enough water to cover salmon and bring to a boil. Reduce the heat to a simmer. Place six slices of salmon in the pan and poach for 30 seconds; remove with a slotted spoon and transfer to a plate with a paper towel to drain. Repeat until all the salmon is cooked.

4. Place fish slices on a dry plate in a single layer and season them with ⅛ teaspoon of the salt and 1 teaspoon of the sesame oil. Squeeze half the lemon over the slices.

5. After the seaweed is finished soaking, drain and toss with vinegar, the remaining sesame oil, green onion, cucumber, and mushrooms.

6. Dress avocado with juice from the remaining half lemon and remaining ⅛ teaspoon salt.

7. To serve, top the seaweed salad with the salmon and avocado slices.

Per serving: 394 calories; 3.6 g saturated fat; 247 mg sodium; 3 g fiber

Baked Penne Pasta with Shrimp

Serves 4   Prep time: 15 minutes   Total time: 1 hour 5 minutes

2 cups whole grain penne pasta (about 5.32 ounces)

Vegetable oil cooking spray

1 large onion, finely sliced

4 cloves garlic, finely minced

2 sweet red peppers, sliced

½ teaspoon salt

3 tomatoes, chopped

2 cups chopped chard

2 tablespoons chopped fresh oregano

1 tablespoon chopped fresh rosemary

1 tablespoon olive oil

1½ pounds shrimp, shelled and deveined

1. Preheat oven to 375 degrees.

2. Prepare the pasta according to package directions.

3. Heat a large ovenproof skillet over medium heat. Spray with cooking oil spray and add onion and half the garlic to skillet. Cook, stirring regularly, for 3 minutes. Add red peppers and cook for 5 more minutes. Remove from heat.

4. In a large bowl combine salt, tomatoes, chard, oregano, rosemary, red pepper mixture, olive oil and the cooked pasta.

5. Place in a baking dish, cover with foil, and bake for 20 minutes. Remove foil and bake for an additional 10 minutes.

6. During the last 10 minutes of the pasta baking, toss shrimp in a bowl with the remaining garlic. Coat with vegetable oil spray. Place the shrimp on a baking tray and bake in the oven until just pink, about 6 minutes.

7. To serve, divide pasta into 4 portions and top each portion with a quarter of the shrimp.

Per serving: 406 calories; 1.2 g saturated fat; 590 mg sodium; 8 g fiber

CREAMY MAC AND NO CHEESE

Serves 4   Prep time: 10 minutes   Total time: 45 minutes

½ pound whole grain macaroni	½ teaspoon mustard powder
1½ cups chopped cauliflower	½ teaspoon paprika
1 cup roasted winter squash (fresh or frozen)	¼ teaspoon salt
	Black pepper, to taste
3 tablespoons chopped cashews	3 Wasa whole grain crispbreads, pulverized
1 tablespoon Bestlife spread	

1. Preheat oven to 375 degrees.

2. Cook macaroni according to package directions. Drain and set aside in a large mixing bowl.

3. Place cauliflower in a medium-size pot. Cover with water and bring to a boil. Reduce to a simmer and cook until tender, about 10 minutes.

4. Drain cauliflower, reserving ½ cup of cooking water. Puree cauliflower, squash, cashews, Bestlife spread, reserved cooking water, mustard powder, paprika, and salt in a blender until very smooth, about 1 minute.

5. Combine the macaroni and cauliflower mixture and mix well. Transfer the mixture to a 9-inch ovenproof skillet. Top with black pepper and pulverized crispbreads.

6. Bake for 10 minutes. Turn oven to a broil and cook until top is browned, about 5 minutes. Serve immediately.

Per serving: 319 calories; 1.2 g saturated fat; 243 mg sodium; 10 g fiber

TOFU VEGETABLE SOUP WITH KOMBU

Serves 4   Prep time: 15 minutes   Total time: 50 minutes

Vegetable oil cooking spray	1 teaspoon low-sodium soy sauce
3 cloves garlic, minced	1 ounce kombu
1 onion, finely sliced	16 ounces firm tofu, cut into cubes
1 teaspoon grated fresh ginger	Leaves of 1 small head or ½ large head bok choy
1 tablespoon miso paste	
6 cups water	1 cup sliced shiitake mushrooms

1. Heat a heavy-bottom soup pot over medium heat. Spray with vegetable oil spray, add garlic, onion, and ginger. Stir constantly for 3 minutes. Add miso and slowly add water, taking care to dissolve the miso. Once the miso is dissolved, add the remaining water, soy sauce, and kombu.

2. Bring soup to a boil, reduce heat, and simmer for 20 minutes. Add tofu, bok choy, and shiitake mushrooms, then simmer for an additional 10 minutes. Serve hot.

Per serving: 284 calories; 1.7 g saturated fat; 408 mg sodium; 8 g fiber

Whole Grain Thin Spaghetti with Peanut Sauce

Serves 4   Prep time: 5 minutes   Total time: 15 minutes

2 tablespoons peanut butter

1 tablespoon white vinegar

1 tablespoon water

4 ounces thin whole grain spaghetti
cooked according to package directions

1 cup shredded carrots

¼ cup fresh cilantro

1. In a large bowl, combine peanut butter, vinegar, and water until smooth.

2. Add spaghetti, carrots, and cilantro to peanut butter mixture, toss, and serve.

Per serving: 158 calories; .9 g saturated fat; 59 mg sodium; 1 g fiber

Veggie Chili with Kale

*Serves 4   Prep time: 10 minutes   Total time: 50 minutes (plus at least
3 hours for tofu to freeze and then thaw)*

Vegetable oil spray

1 large onion, chopped

3 cloves garlic, minced

8 ounces firm or very firm tofu,
drained thoroughly, frozen solid
and defrosted

6 cups water

3 tomatoes, chopped, or 3 cups
canned, no salt added, chopped

2 sweet red peppers, seeds removed,
finely chopped

2 carrots, chopped

⅛ teaspoon cayenne, or more
to taste

2 tablespoons chili powder

1½ cups cooked red kidney beans
(dried or canned, no salt added,
drained and rinsed)

2 cups finely chopped kale

¼ teaspoon salt

1. Heat large heavy-bottom stockpot over medium heat. Coat with
vegetable oil spray, add onion and garlic, and cook until brown, stirring
regularly, about 5 minutes.

2. Crumble thawed tofu, which will be similar to the consistency of
ground beef. Add to the onion mixture. Continue cooking, stirring
regularly, for 5 minutes.

3. Add water, tomatoes, red peppers, carrots, cayenne, chili powder, kidney beans, and kale. Stir and bring to a boil.

4. Reduce heat and simmer for 30 minutes. Stir in salt. Serve hot.

Per serving: 324 calories; 1.6 g saturated fat; 434 mg sodium; 18 g fiber

POLENTA

Serves 4   Prep time: 5 minutes   Total time: 25 minutes

Vegetable oil spray	1½ tablespoons olive oil
3 cups water	One large pinch salt
1 cup cornmeal	

1. Preheat oven to 350 degrees. Spray a 9 × 9-inch baking pan with vegetable oil spray.

2. Bring water to a boil in a medium-size pan. Slowly add cornmeal, stirring continuously to avoid lumps.

3. Reduce heat to medium and continue to cook, stirring, for 5 minutes. Remove from heat and stir in olive oil and salt.

4. Pour cornmeal mixture into baking pan and cook for 10 minutes. Turn oven to broil and cook until top is browned, about 5 more minutes.

Per serving: 202 calories; 1.2 g saturated fat; 42 mg sodium; 4 g fiber

Snack

ACAI POPSICLE

Serves 4   Prep time: 5 minutes   Total time: 3 hours (includes freezing time)

1 cup frozen acai puree, defrosted

5 cups skim milk

2 tablespoons honey

1. Place all the ingredients into a blender and blend until smooth, about 1 minute.

2. Pour the mixture into four Popsicle molds or paper cups. Place a popsicle stick or chopstick in the middle of each cup and freeze for 3 hours or until solid.

3. To serve, remove from molds or peel away the paper cup. Extra popsicles can be stored in the freezer for future snacks.

Per serving: 155 calories; .5 g saturated fat; 132 mg sodium; 1 g fiber

Treat

ZUCCHINI OLIVE OIL CAKE

Serves 8   Prep time: 10 minutes   Total time: 30 minutes

1 egg	Pinch ground cloves
¼ cup olive oil	Pinch ground ginger
⅓ cup sugar	Pinch grated nutmeg
¼ cup whole wheat flour	½ cup shredded zucchini
½ teaspoon baking soda	6 tablespoons chopped walnuts
½ teaspoon low-sodium baking powder	Vegetable oil cooking spray
½ teaspoon cinnamon	

1. Preheat oven to 350 degrees. Combine all the ingredients except vegetable oil spray in a mixer and mix until just fully incorporated.

2. Spray a 9-inch pie plate with vegetable oil spray. Pour batter into pie plate and spread to evenly coat the plate.

3. Bake until the cake is slightly springy to the touch and tests clean with a knife, about 20 minutes. Slice and serve. Extra portions can be frozen for future treats.

Per serving: 155 calories; 1.5 g saturated fat; 89 mg sodium; 1 g fiber

BAKED APPLE

Serves 4   Prep time: 5 minutes   Total time: 25 minutes

Vegetable oil cooking spray

4 apples, halved, core removed

4 teaspoons olive oil

2 tablespoons brown sugar

½ teaspoon ground cinnamon

2 tablespoons low-fat sour cream

1. Preheat oven to 325 degrees. Spray a baking dish with vegetable oil.

2. In a large bowl, toss apples with olive oil, brown sugar, and cinnamon.

3. Place apples in the baking dish skin-side up. Top the apples with any sugar that remains in the bowl. Bake until tender, about 20 minutes. Serve warm, room temperature, or cold topped with sour cream.

Per serving: 153 calories; 1.3 g saturated fat; 9 mg sodium; 3 g fiber

CHOCOLATE SESAME BISCOTTI

Serves 6   Prep time: 10 minutes   Total time: 30 minutes

3 tablespoons pureed silken tofu

¼ cup sugar plus 1 teaspoon for rolling

1 teaspoon baking powder

2 tablespoons sesame oil

¼ cup plus 2 tablespoons flour

2 tablespoons cocoa powder

¼ cup whole wheat flour

2 tablespoons sesame seeds

1. Preheat oven to 375 degrees.

2. In food processor combine all the ingredients except the teaspoon sugar, and process for 1 minute.

3. Remove dough, sprinkle with the teaspoon sugar, and roll into a log 1 inch in diameter. Place on baking sheet and bake for 10 minutes. Remove from oven, let cool for 5 minutes, and slice into ½-inch slices (there should be about 12 large or 18 small cookies). Return slices to pan and place them in the oven. Turn the oven off and let biscotti dry for 15 minutes or overnight before serving. The longer you dry biscotti, the harder the cookies will be.

Per serving: 149 calories; 1 g saturated fat; 84 mg sodium; 2 g fiber

Carrot Oatmeal Cookie

Serves 6   Prep time: 5 minutes   Total time: 15 minutes

1 cup rolled oats

2 tablespoons olive oil

2 tablespoons soy or skim milk

1 tablespoon sugar

1 tablespoon honey

¼ cup shredded carrot

1 tablespoon currants

¼ cup chopped walnuts

½ teaspoon baking powder

Pinch salt

Vegetable oil cooking spray

1. Preheat oven to 350 degrees.

2. Combine all but the oil spray; process for 2 minutes.

3. Spray a cookie sheet with oil spray. Divide batter into 6 cookies. Flatten and bake till golden, about 7 minutes.

Per serving: 150 calories; 1.1 g saturated fat; 73 mg sodium; 2 g fiber

Stuffed Baked Peach

Serves 1   Prep time: 5 minutes   Total time: 20 minutes

2 tablespoons nonfat ricotta

1 teaspoon honey

Dash of vanilla extract

1 peach, pit removed, halved

1 teaspoon finely chopped almonds

1. Preheat oven to 375 degrees.

2. In a small bowl combine ricotta, honey, and vanilla. Stuff peach halves with ricotta mixture and place on a baking sheet.

3. Bake for 15 minutes. Top with almonds and serve warm or cool.

Per serving: 148 calories; .5 g saturated fat; 75 mg sodium; 3 g fiber

CHAPTER 8

Putting It All Together

THE KEY TO INCORPORATING REGULAR EXERCISE, healthy eating, effective skin care, and good sleep habits into your life is all about being organized and efficient. To show you what I mean by that, here's what a week in the lives of four different people looks like. One person hasn't committed to much physical activity (we'll call her Pre–Level I) and is eating 1,500 calories; one is a Level I exerciser eating 1,700 calories; one is a Level II exerciser eating 2,000 calories; and one is a Level III exerciser eating 2,500 calories.

PRE-LEVEL I, 1,500 CALORIES

This schedule isn't difficult to follow and leaves plenty of room for more exercise, should you decide to step up your physical activity.

Monday

7:00 A.M.

Wake up

7:15 A.M.

Physical activity: Stretches and core strengtheners

7:30 A.M.

Skin care: Cleanse, nourish, sunscreen

7:45 A.M.

Breakfast: Yogurt Pomegranate Parfait; English muffin with Bestlife spread

12:30 P.M.

Lunch: Couscous Peach Salad; Quick Roasted Kale

3:00 P.M.

Snack: Grape, Cardamom, and Yogurt Parfait

6:30 P.M.

Dinner: Creamy Mac and No Cheese; Tomato Salad; Steamed Broccoli with Garlic

10:45 P.M.

Skin care: Polish, cleanse, nourish

11:00 P.M.

Sleep

Tuesday

7:00 A.M.

Wake up

7:15 A.M.

Physical activity: Stretches and core strengtheners

7:30 A.M.

Skin care: Cleanse, nourish, sunscreen

7:45 A.M.

Breakfast: Tofu Scramble; mango and blackberries

12:30 P.M.

Lunch: Open Face Almond Butter Sandwich; Celery Salad

3:00 P.M.

Snack: Green tea with soy milk

6:30 P.M.

Dinner: Salmon Salad with Avocado, Hijiki, Cucumber, and Mushrooms; black rice; grapefruit and raspberries

10:45 P.M.

Skin care: Polish, cleanse, nourish

11:00 P.M.

Sleep

Wednesday

7:00 A.M.

Wake up

7:15 A.M.

Physical activity: Stretches and core strengtheners

7:30 A.M.

Skin care: Cleanse, nourish, sunscreen

7:45 A.M.

Breakfast: Egg White and Spinach Omelet; Wasa multigrain crispbread; blackberries and honey; skim milk

12:30 P.M.

Lunch: Portobello Sandwich; plum salad with pistachios; baby carrots and tahini

3:00 P.M.

Snack: Chocolate Ginger Latte

6:30 P.M.

Dinner: Tofu Vegetable Soup with Kombu; Whole Grain Thin Spaghetti with Peanut Sauce; orange

10:45 P.M.

Skin care: Polish, cleanse, nourish.

11:00 P.M.

Sleep

Thursday

7:00 A.M.

Wake up

7:15 A.M.

Physical activity: Stretches and core strengtheners

7:30 A.M.

Skin care: Cleanse, nourish, sunscreen

7:45 A.M.

Breakfast: Whole Grain Cream of Wheat; skim milk

12:30 P.M.

Lunch: Sesame Shrimp Salad with Napa Cabbage and Bean Sprouts; blueberries and nonfat plain yogurt

3:00 P.M.

Snack: Grape, Cinnamon, and Yogurt Parfait

6:30 P.M.

Dinner: Veggie Chili; Polenta

10:45 P.M.

Skin care: Polish, cleanse, nourish

11:00 P.M.

Sleep

Friday

7:00 A.M.

Wake up

7:15 A.M.

Physical activity: Stretches and core strengtheners

7:30 A.M.

Skin care: Cleanse, nourish, sunscreen

7:45 A.M.

Breakfast: Oatmeal with soy milk, strawberries, and slivered almonds

12:30 P.M.

Lunch: Tempeh, Lettuce, and Tomato Sandwich

3:00 P.M.

Snack: Cucumber with Ricotta Dip

6:30 P.M.

Dinner: Poached Chicken Curry; brown rice

10:45 P.M.

Skin care: Polish, cleanse, nourish

12:00 A.M.

Sleep

Saturday

8:00 A.M.

Wake up

8:15 A.M.

Physical activity:

Stretches and core strengtheners

20-minute walk

9:00 A.M.

Skin care: Cleanse, nourish, sunscreen

9:15 A.M.

Breakfast: Whole grain flake cereal, sunflower seeds, blackberries, and soy milk

1:00 P.M.

Lunch: Tuna Salad; strawberries; Wasa multigrain crispbread

4:00 P.M.

Snack: Mango Smoothie

7:30 P.M.

Dinner: Pork Loin with Turnips, Apples, and Onions; barley and arugula

11:45 P.M.

Skin care: Polish, cleanse, nourish

12:00 A.M.

Sleep

Sunday

8:00 A.M.

Wake up

8:15 A.M.

Physical activity:

Stretches and core strengtheners

20-minute walk

9:00 A.M.

Skin care: Cleanse, nourish, sunscreen

9:15 A.M.

Breakfast: Blueberry Oatmeal Pancakes; calcium-fortified orange juice

1:00 P.M.

Lunch: Black Bean Salad; Garlic Toast; orange

3:00 P.M.

Snack: Carrots with Spiced Yogurt Dip

6:30 P.M.

Dinner: Baked Penne Pasta with Shrimp; Arugula and Fennel Salad

10:45 P.M.

Skin care: Polish, cleanse, nourish

11:00 P.M.

Sleep

LEVEL I, 1,700 CALORIES

This is the perfect schedule for anyone with a busy week. You can get most of your cardio in on the weekends.

Monday

6:00 A.M.

Wake up

6:15 A.M.

Physical activity:

Stretches and core strengtheners

Strength training

6:45 A.M.

Skin care: Cleanse, nourish, sunscreen

7:00 A.M.

Breakfast: Acai Almond Butter Smoothie with whole grain cereal

12:30 P.M.

Lunch: Sardine Salad; whole wheat roll with olive oil; grapes and figs

1:00 P.M.

Physical activity: 20-minute walk

3:00 P.M.

Snack: Fresh Mint Tea with honey

6:30 P.M.

Dinner: Baked Eggplant with Ground Turkey; cracked wheat; baby spinach; cantaloupe

Treat: Graham Cracker with Banana and Walnuts

9:45 P.M.

Skin care: Polish, cleanse, nourish

10:00 P.M.

Sleep

Tuesday

6:00 A.M.

Wake up

6:15 A.M.

Physical activity: Stretches and core strengtheners

6:45 A.M.

Skin care: Cleanse, nourish, sunscreen

7:00 A.M.

Breakfast: Muesli with skim milk, blackberries, and almonds

12:30 P.M.

Lunch: Chicken, Grapefruit, and Arugula Salad; two Wasa multigrain crispbreads with Bestlife spread

1:00 P.M.

Physical activity: 20-minute walk

3:00 P.M.

Snack: Pomegranate Freeze

6:30 P.M.

Dinner: Poached Trout with Tomato and Basil; Spicy Farro with Mint and Parsley; strawberries

Treat: Zucchini Olive Oil Cake

9:45 P.M.

Skin care: Polish, cleanse, nourish

10:00 P.M.

Sleep

Wednesday

6:00 A.M.

Wake up

6:15 A.M.

Physical activity:

Stretches and core strengtheners

Strength training

6:45 A.M.

Skin care: Cleanse, nourish, sunscreen

7:00 A.M.

Breakfast: Shredded wheat with flaxseed, walnuts, strawberries, and soy milk

12:30 P.M.

Lunch: Edamame Dip; brown rice cakes; Cabbage Salad; honeydew melon

3:00 P.M.

Snack: Acai Popsicle

6:30 P.M.

Dinner: Braised Chicken Legs in Red Wine with Lentils, Fennel, and Kale; mixed greens with mushrooms and olive oil–lemon dressing; blueberries

Treat: Air-popped popcorn

9:45 P.M.

Skin care: Polish, cleanse, nourish.

10:00 P.M.

Sleep

Thursday

6:00 A.M.

Wake up

6:15 A.M.

Physical activity: Stretches and core strengtheners

6:45 A.M.

Skin care: Cleanse, nourish, sunscreen

7:00 A.M.

Breakfast: Irish oatmeal with dried apricots, almonds, and skim milk

12:30 P.M.

Lunch: Salmon and avocado sushi roll; pineapple and walnuts

1:00 P.M.

Physical activity: 20-minute walk

3:00 P.M.

Snack: Nonfat yogurt with raspberries, cashews, and graham cracker

6:30 P.M.

Dinner: Slow Cooked Lamb with Tomato, Cauliflower, and Chard; Whole Grain Crostini; orange

Treat: Banana with dark chocolate chips and pine nuts

9:45 P.M.

Skin care: Polish, cleanse, nourish

10:00 P.M.

Sleep

Friday

6:00 A.M.

Wake up

6:15 A.M.

Physical activity:

Stretches and core strengtheners

Strength training

6:45 A.M.

Skin care: Cleanse, nourish, sunscreen

7:00 A.M.

Breakfast: Blackberry Smoothie

12:30 P.M.

Lunch: Lentil soup with Parmesan cheese and baby spinach; Wasa multigrain crispbread; grapefruit and pistachios

1:00 P.M.

Physical activity: 20-minute walk

3:00 P.M.

Snack: Acai Popsicle

6:30 P.M.

Dinner: Spiced Cod; Cracked Wheat Salad

Treat: Pretzels, Golden Raisins, and Dark Chocolate Trail Mix

10:45 P.M.

Skin care: Polish, cleanse, nourish

11:00 P.M.

Sleep

Saturday

7:00 A.M.

Wake up

7:15 A.M.

Physical activity:

Stretches and core strengtheners

1-hour walk

8:30 A.M.

Skin care: Cleanse, nourish, sunscreen

8:45 A.M.

Breakfast: Yogurt Parfait

1:00 P.M.

Lunch: Cannellini Bean Spread on Whole Grain Pita; Arugula Salad; honeydew melon

3:00 P.M.

Physical activity: Tennis

4:00 P.M.

Snack: Strawberry Milk

7:30 P.M.

Dinner: Sweet Potato and Turkey Shepherd's Pie; Coleslaw with Mustard Vinaigrette; whole wheat roll with olive oil; raspberries

Treat: Baked Apple

10:45 P.M.

Skin care: Polish, cleanse, nourish

11:00 P.M.

Sleep

Sunday

7:00 A.M.

Wake up

7:15 A.M.

Physical activity:

Stretches and core strengtheners

1-hour walk

8:30 A.M.

Skin care: Cleanse, nourish, sunscreen

8:45 A.M.

Breakfast: Banana Spice Smoothie; Wasa multigrain crispbread and peanut butter

1:00 P.M.

Lunch: Goat Cheese Sandwich; Citrus Salad

3:00 P.M.

Snack: Cucumber with Yogurt Dip

6:30 P.M.

Dinner: Trout Gumbo; Mixed Baby Green Salad; raspberries

Treat: Dark chocolate sorbet

9:45 P.M.

Skin care: Polish, cleanse, nourish

10:00 P.M.

Sleep

LEVEL II, 2,000 CALORIES

If you prefer to get your cardio in at night, this is a good plan for you.

Monday

6:00 A.M.

Wake up

6:15 A.M.

Physical activity: Stretches and core strengtheners

6:45 A.M.

Skin care: Cleanse, nourish, sunscreen

7:30 A.M.

Breakfast: Yogurt Pomegranate Parfait; English muffin with Bestlife spread

12:30 P.M.

Lunch: Couscous Peach Salad; Quick Roasted Kale

3:00 P.M.

Snack: Grape, Cardamom, and Yogurt Parfait

5:00 P.M.

Physical activity:

45 minutes on the elliptical trainer

Strength training

6:30 P.M.

Dinner: Creamy Mac and No Cheese; Tomato Salad; Steamed Broccoli with Garlic and olive oil

Treat: Chocolate Sesame Biscotti with almond butter

9:45 P.M.

Skin care: Polish, cleanse, nourish

10:00 P.M.

Sleep

Tuesday

6:00 A.M.

Wake up

6:15 A.M.

Physical activity: Stretches and core strengtheners

6:45 A.M.

Skin care: Cleanse, nourish, sunscreen

7:30 A.M.

Breakfast: Tofu Scramble; mango and blackberries

12:30 P.M.

Lunch: Almond Butter Sandwich; Celery Salad

3:00 P.M.

Snack: Green tea with soy milk

5:00 P.M.

45-minute walk

6:30 P.M.

Dinner: Salmon Salad with Avocado, Hijiki, Cucumber, and Mushrooms; black rice; grapefruit and walnuts

Treat: Poached Pear with pecans

9:45 P.M.

Skin care: Polish, cleanse, nourish

10:00 P.M.

Sleep

Wednesday

6:00 A.M.

Wake up

6:15 A.M.

Physical activity:

Stretches and core strengtheners

Strength training

6:45 A.M.

Skin care: Cleanse, nourish, sunscreen

7:30 A.M.

Breakfast: Egg White and Spinach Omelet; Wasa multigrain crispbread; blackberries and honey; skim milk

12:30 P.M.

Lunch: Portobello Sandwich; plum salad with pistachios; baby carrots and tahini

3:00 P.M.

Snack: Chocolate Ginger Latte

6:30 P.M.

Dinner: Tofu Vegetable Soup with Kombu; Whole Grain Thin Spaghetti with Peanut Sauce; orange; Wasa multigrain crispbreads with Bestlife spread

Treat: Orange with Spices and Pecans

8:00 P.M.

Physical activity: Darts

9:45 P.M.

Skin care: Polish, cleanse, nourish

10:00 P.M.

Sleep

Thursday

6:00 A.M.

Wake up

6:15 A.M.

Physical activity: Stretches and core strengtheners

6:45 A.M.

Skin care: Cleanse, nourish, sunscreen

7:30 A.M.

Breakfast: Whole Grain Cream of Wheat; skim milk

12:30 P.M.

Lunch: Sesame Shrimp Salad with Napa Cabbage and Bean Sprouts; brown rice cakes with avocado; blueberries and nonfat plain yogurt

3:00 P.M.

Snack: Grape, Cinnamon, and Yogurt Parfait

5:00 P.M.

Physical activity: 45-minute walk

6:30 P.M.

Dinner: Veggie Chili; Polenta with reduced-fat cheddar cheese; mixed baby greens salad

Treat: Dark chocolate with fresh strawberries and pecans

9:45 P.M.

Skin care: Polish, cleanse, nourish

10:00 P.M.

Sleep

Friday

6:00 A.M.

Wake up

6:15 A.M.

Physical activity: Stretches and core strengtheners

6:45 A.M.

Skin care: Cleanse, nourish, sunscreen

7:30 A.M.

Breakfast: Oatmeal with soy milk, strawberries, and slivered almonds

12:30 P.M.

Lunch: Tempeh, Lettuce, and Tomato Sandwich; spinach salad

3:00 P.M.

Snack: Cucumber with Ricotta Dip

5:00 P.M.

Physical activity:

45 minutes on the elliptical trainer

Strength training

6:30 P.M.

Dinner: Poached Chicken Curry; brown rice; Spicy Mango Relish

Treat: Carrot Oatmeal Cookie with almond butter

10:45 P.M.

Skin care: Polish, cleanse, nourish

11:00 P.M.

Sleep

Saturday

7:00 A.M.

Wake up

7:15 A.M.

Physical activity:

Stretches and core strengtheners

1 hour cycling

8:45 A.M.

Skin care: Cleanse, nourish, sunscreen

9:00 A.M.

Breakfast: Whole grain flake cereal and shredded wheat, sunflower seeds, blackberries, and soy milk

1:00 P.M.

Lunch: Tuna Salad; whole wheat roll; strawberries

3:00 P.M.

Physical activity: In-line skating

4:00 P.M.

Snack: Mango Smoothie

7:30 P.M.

Dinner: Pork Loin with Turnips, Apples, and Onions; barley, pecans, and arugula

Treat: Stuffed Baked Peach and nonfat Greek yogurt

10:45 P.M.

Skin care: Polish, cleanse, nourish

11:00 P.M.

Sleep

Sunday

7:00 A.M.

Wake up

7:15 A.M.

Physical activity:

Stretches and core strengtheners

1 hour cycling

8:45 A.M.

Skin care: Cleanse, nourish, sunscreen

9:00 A.M.

Breakfast: Blueberry Oatmeal Pancakes topped with blueberries and walnuts; calcium-fortified orange juice

1:00 P.M.

Lunch: Black Bean Salad; Garlic Toast; orange

3:00 P.M.

Snack: Carrots with Spiced Yogurt Dip

6:30 P.M.

Dinner: Baked Penne Pasta with Shrimp; Arugula and Fennel Salad

Treat: Trail mix

9:45 P.M.

Skin care: Polish, cleanse, nourish

10:00 P.M.

Sleep

LEVEL III, 2,500 CALORIES

This is just one example of how to get a substantial amount of exercise in each day. Most people find that they have to get up pretty early to reach their daily goal.

Monday

5:30 A.M.

Wake up

5:45 A.M.

Physical activity:

Stretches and core strengtheners

1-hour run

7:00 A.M.

Skin care: Cleanse, nourish, sunscreen

7:15 A.M.

Breakfast: Acai Almond Butter Smoothie with whole grain cereal

10 A.M.

Snack: Apple with sunflower seed butter

12:30 P.M.

Lunch: Sardine Salad; whole wheat roll with olive oil; grapes, figs, and pecans

3:00 P.M.

Snack: Fresh Mint Tea

6:30 P.M.

Dinner: Baked Eggplant with Ground Turkey; cracked wheat; baby spinach; and cantaloupe

Treat: Graham Cracker with Banana and Walnuts

9:15 P.M.

Skin care: Polish, cleanse, nourish

9:30 P.M.

Sleep

Tuesday

5:30 A.M.

Wake up

5:45 A.M.

Physical activity:

Stretches and core strengtheners

Strength training

1-hour swim

7:15 A.M.

Skin care: Cleanse, nourish, sunscreen

7:30 A.M.

Breakfast: Muesli with skim milk, blackberries, and almonds

10 A.M.

Snack: Whole wheat pita with almond butter

12:30 P.M.

Lunch: Chicken, Grapefruit and Arugula Salad; 2 Wasa multigrain crackers with Bestlife spread

3:00 P.M.

Snack: Pomegranate Freeze

6:30 P.M.

Dinner: Poached Trout with Tomato and Basil; Spicy Farro with Mint and Parsley; strawberries

Treat: Zucchini Olive Oil Cake with applesauce

9:15 P.M.

Skin care: Polish, cleanse, nourish

9:30 P.M.

Sleep

Wednesday

5:30 A.M.

Wake up

5:45 A.M.

Physical activity: Stretches and core strengtheners

6:00 A.M.

Skin care: Cleanse, nourish, sunscreen

6:15 A.M.

Breakfast: Shredded wheat with flaxseed, walnuts, strawberries, and soy milk

10:00 A.M.

Snack: Trail mix

12:30 P.M.

Lunch: Edamame Dip; brown rice cakes; Cabbage Salad; honeydew melon and slivered almonds

3:00 P.M.

Snack: Acai Popsicle

5:00 P.M.

Physical activity: Squash

6:30 P.M.

Dinner: Braised Chicken Legs in Red Wine with Lentils, Fennel, and Kale; mixed greens with mushrooms and olive oil-lemon dressing; whole wheat rolls; blueberries

Treat: Air-popped popcorn

9:15 P.M.

Skin care: Polish, cleanse, nourish

9:30 P.M.

Sleep

Thursday

5:30 A.M.

Wake up

5:45 A.M.

Physical activity:

Stretches and core strengtheners

Strength training

1-hour run

7:15 A.M.

Skin care: Cleanse, nourish, sunscreen

7:30 A.M.

Breakfast: Irish oatmeal with dried apricots, almonds, and skim milk

10:00 A.M.

Snack: 2 Wasa multigrain crispbreads with mozzarella and tomato; grapes

12:30 P.M.

Lunch: Salmon and avocado sushi roll; pineapple and walnuts

3:00 P.M.

Snack: Nonfat yogurt with raspberries, cashews, and graham cracker

6:30 P.M.

Dinner: Slow Cooked Lamb with Tomato, Cauliflower, and Chard; Whole Grain Crostini; orange, blueberries, and macadamia nuts

Treat: Banana and pear with dark chocolate chips and pine nuts

9:15 P.M.

Skin care: Polish, cleanse, nourish

9:30 P.M.

Sleep

Friday

5:30 A.M.

Wake up

5:45 A.M.

Physical activity:

Stretches and core strengtheners

1-hour swim

7:00 A.M.

Skin care: Cleanse, nourish, sunscreen

7:15 A.M.

Breakfast: Blackberry Smoothie

10:00 A.M.

Snack: Whole wheat pita with sunflower seed butter

12:30 P.M.

Lunch: Lentil Soup with Parmesan cheese and baby spinach; Wasa multigrain crispbreads; grapefruit, honey, and pistachios

3:00 P.M.

Snack: Acai Popsicle

6:30 P.M.

Dinner: Spiced Cod; Cracked Wheat Salad

Treat: Pretzels, Golden Raisins, and Dark Chocolate Trail Mix

10:15 P.M.

Skin care: Polish, cleanse, nourish

10:30 P.M.

Sleep

Saturday

6:30 A.M.

Wake up

6:45 A.M.

Physical activity:

Stretches and core strengtheners

Half of the strength training routine

80-minute run

8:30 A.M.

Skin care: Cleanse, nourish, sunscreen

8:45 A.M.

Breakfast: Yogurt Parfait

11:00 A.M.

Snack: Pear with almond butter

1:00 P.M.

Lunch: Cannellini Bean Spread on Whole Grain Pita; Arugula Salad; honeydew melon and pistachios

3:00 P.M.

Physical activity: Tennis

4:00 P.M.

Snack: Strawberry Milk

7:30 P.M.

Dinner: Sweet Potato and Turkey Shepherd's Pie; Coleslaw with Mustard Vinaigrette; whole wheat roll with olive oil; raspberries with honey and pomegranate seeds.

Treat: Baked Apple with low-fat caramel sauce and pecans

10:45 P.M.

Skin care: Polish, cleanse, nourish

11:00 P.M.

Sleep

Sunday

6:30 A.M.

Wake up

6:45 A.M.

Physical activity:

Stretches and core strengtheners

Other half of the strength training routine

80 minutes of cycling

8:30 A.M.

Skin care: Cleanse, nourish, sunscreen

8:45 A.M.

Breakfast: Banana Spice Smoothie; Wasa multigrain crispbread and peanut butter

11:00 A.M.

Snack: Wasa multigrain crispbreads with peanut butter, celery, and honey

1:00 P.M.

Lunch: Goat Cheese Sandwich; Citrus Salad with grapes and maple syrup

3:00 P.M.

Physical activity: Ping-Pong

4:00 P.M.

Snack: Cucumber with Yogurt Dip

6:30 P.M.

Dinner: Trout Gumbo; Mixed Baby Green Salad; brown rice; raspberries

Treat: Dark chocolate sorbet with pecans

9:15 P.M.

Skin care: Polish, cleanse, nourish

9:30 P.M.

Sleep

Acknowledgments

WITH SPECIAL THANKS to Daryn Eller, Janis Jibrin, RD, Donna Fennessy, Sidra Forman, Molly Borman-Pullen, Michelle Kennedy, and Tracy Gensler for their excellent contributions to this book. Thanks, too, to Angeli Lacson for helping to facilitate this project. We're also very grateful for the insights from all of the researchers quoted throughout this book.

Index